THE
WINTER
WONDER
DIET

The
WINTER WONDER
Diet

The balanced 18-day plan
for *real* weight loss

Bronwen Meredith

Roger Houghton
London

First published 1986
© Bronwen Meredith 1986
Illustrations © Roger Houghton Ltd 1986

Set in Bembo Roman by Gee Graphics Ltd
Printed and bound in Great Britain by Biddles Ltd,
Guildford, Surrey
for Roger Houghton Ltd, in association with
J.M. Dent and Sons Ltd, Aldine House, 33 Welbeck Street,
London W1M 8LX

*Every care has been taken in preparing
these diets and exercises but readers
should have regard to their age and state
of health before undertaking them. If you
are in any doubt, consult your medical
adviser beforehand, as no responsibility
can be accepted by the author or publisher
for any errors or omissions or for any
illness or injury sustained.*

British Library Cataloguing in Publication Data
Meredith, Bronwen
     The winter wonder diet : the balanced 18–day plan for real
     weight loss.
     1. Reducing diets   2. Physical fitness
     I. Title
     6132'5   RM222.2

ISBN 1 85203 004 6

Contents

INTRODUCTION

One fact is clear: dieting is the obsession of the decade, and the number of people constantly preoccupied with losing weight is staggeringly high. It is estimated that about one-third of the adult population of Great Britain is on a diet, or at least about to go on one. But which diet? There are so many theories, so many conflicting views, so many suggestions. The choice is rampant – and so is the confusion. There are protagonists for all protein, for all vegetables, for wholegrains, for pouring in fibre, for only raw food, for limited carbohydrates, for simply eating less (the calorie counters), for grapefruit, for pineapple and so forth. Every diet has its advocates and dissenters. Not all diets have come from medical sources; many ideas from self-styled nutritionists have caught the imagination of the public. What is certain is that there is always some scientific criticism from someone – medicine thrives and develops on such controversy, and disagreement is par for the nutritional course.

It has also become the fashion in some quarters to say that diets don't work and that only a change in the type of food can be effective, combined with a continual programme of energetic exercise. This is all perfectly valid, but only up to a point. It is time that food intake, weight control and the role of exercise be put into sound, sensible perspective.

The majority of overweight people do require the impetus of a limited diet to get them over the first fat hurdle, and the source, quality and quantity of foods are all vital factors. Calories still count when trying to lose weight. If you require more energy than that supplied by food within a twenty-four hour period, the body will burn up stored fat for fuel. The mathematical equation is not so constant nor so reliable when you eat more food than you require for energy. You do not go on adding fat at a set rate for every extra calorie, otherwise almost everybody would be gross – the body has a way of organising a degree of control. And when it comes to exercise, the arguments in favour of such aerobics as jogging or other strenuous routines may be persuasive but there are millions of people who are unconvinced and cannot overcome their natural disinclination for extreme exertion. Indeed, there is a forceful school of medical thought that puts forward the view that man was never really meant to run and puff and pant except in an emergency – otherwise there would be more evidence of it. The current fitness reaction to man's too sedentary life today is at times carried too far.

So what is the answer to combat excess weight and general unhealthiness? One has to look back to man's evolution, and when the facts emerge they might at first glance appear too simple to be credible in our scientifically programmed world. Yet they provide the key to weight control and achieving the body's optimum healthy state. Man lived off vegetation and hunted prey, the latter clearly being an instinctive need for animal flesh of some sort; killing in this way was never just a sport. So an eating pattern became established: hearty – even gluttonous – consumption of freshly caught game during the short period before it became rancid; then, in the interim, subsistence came from the surrounding plants. Man's gut became adjusted accordingly to cope with the digestion at different times of these two metabolically different foods.

In general terms, animal, bird and fish foods require an acid state in the stomach for digestion, while food from vegetation – grains, vegetables, fruits – need an alkaline medium for breakdown and benefit from the vital nutrients. However, many vegetables and fruits and some fats naturally contain the elements that provoke the ideal acid/alkali balance in the digestive system, so they are in essence neutral foods. The biochemical reactions within the body during food assimilation are trigger points for health, and some medical sources believe that there is a greater chance of health equilibrium if the acid and alkaline foods are not combined in one meal.

And now there is evidence that these basic metabolicalprocesses can be manipulated to positively influence weight loss and at the same time cleanse and de-toxify the body. Professor Wolfgang G. Claren has found that patients at the Austrian clinic with which he is associated lose pounds and inches remarkably quickly and healthily if he puts them on his 'swinging diet'. The principle behind the regimen is that when the body is in an accelerated acid state, fat can be burned up faster, and when there is an alkaline medium, toxins are washed away as water is drawn from the cells. Patients are thus put on three days of acid foods, then three days of alkaline foods, for a total of eighteen days.

Why a winter diet? Of course, the diet is equally applicable all year, but because it involves considerable hearty fare it is particularly good news for the winter dieter, who finds the traditional diet food of salads and fruits (and a minimum of everything else) not substantial enough to cope with the rigours of cold weather – a good hot dish is what is often needed. The winter months are an ideal time to lose weight as you can make the cold work for you in many ways. The diet is the crux of it all, and using the framework of Professor Claren's plan, this book presents a detailed programme for eighteen days – the period he recommends as being the most beneficial – and includes many alternative recipes for family meals, plus guides to the most nutritional foods and their value for both health and weight reduction. It's a system which, when combined with realistic exercise, means you can emerge lighter, slimmer, fitter and healthier – benefiting at home from what is being empirically established in the Alpine clinic.

The Clinical View

by Professor Wolfgang G. Claren*

There is no diet in this world which is perfect and right for everyone, whether it is a diet for health maintenance, disease protection or weight control. But there is an unfortunate tendency these days for various dietary regimes to be hailed and publicised as miracle pathways to ultimate health in themselves, without taking into account the countless contributing factors which influence individual metabolism. The real strength and purpose of the diet ideas outlined in this book are the way in which they provide an opportunity for the dieter to experience the tastes and effects of different food groups. It is very necessary to be aware of the body's response to food over and above the feeling of well-being it engenders.

The nutritional ideas behind the eating pattern described in this book are presented in simple, lay terms. It contains a straightforward explanation of the processes of biochemistry which have evolved thoughout the ages and developed into our present digestive system. To the medically trained mind this is but skimming the surface of modern nutritional knowledge, for we now have such a clear understanding of the breakdown patterns of food that our knowledge would fill many volumes. For the surgeon, the study of body fluids has always been highly significant, while for the biochemist this knowledge, together with meticulous and precise study of digestion during the last few decades, has provided a well-defined groundwork for establishing the connection between malnutrition and disease. And through the media, the lay person has thus been alerted to the dangers of bad eating habits and to the benefits of becoming more food conscious.

*The principles behind *The Winter Wonder Diet* are based on published papers and articles presented at international conferences by Professor Claren between 1962 and 1978, under the general heading of 'The Swinging Diet', and researched under the control of the International Institute for Age Therapy.

It is no coincidence that the healthy food revival is happening at a time when new insight is being brought to bear on the elusive aspects of the human ageing process. Research has given birth to a new medical speciality, gerontology, and it is now established that the theoretical lifespan of mankind could be as long as 120 years, were it not for terrestial pollution, cosmic radiation and the general wear and tear of living.

Man has conquered a great many of the ills of bad hygiene and environment, but until recently we have rarely thought about the effects of diet; over the past century we have emphasised and appreciated the finesse and creation of dishes rather than the health value of nutrition – and this is quite apart from the way in which we have blindly accepted processed foods. Modern man had been satisfied with his feeling of well-being – hardly thinking of the hangover as long as the party calls. But now we know that in order to lead a longer, healthier life, we have to give food more serious thought. There is, however, a new danger: that we fall prey to the absolute teachings. Many diets originated as 'cures' under a traditional, clinical regimen and as such proved to be worthy corrective aids, but it is unrealistic and impractical to consider them as lifetime guides.

A change to fresh and unrefined foods, cutting down on animal fat and keeping the body abundantly supplied with green vegetables and grains which provide the vital minerals and vitamins will set you on the regeneration road to health – this does not involve a radical dietary switch.

As a trained researcher and gerontologist, I realised early in my career, three decades ago, that it was necessary to meticulously decode the eating habits of each individual patient. Analysed in the laboratory, the results led me to the development of the acid–alkaline Swinging Diet and its therapeutic application. It was but one part of interrelated therapies in the treatment of the maladies related to the ageing process. The application of the Diet showed that not only did patients easily and beneficially adjust to a new balance of eating, but they could also, if this involved certain quantity restrictions over the specified time of eighteen days, safely lose weight and give the body a metabolic boost.

Chapter 1

Fat and the Cold

We all know from experience that we tend to put on weight during the winter months and, what is more, we are brought up to justify it as being a necessary and sensible thing in order to combat the cold. Our mothers told us to wrap up well and eat heartily – but how valid is this? In the light of our bio-chemical knowledge of body metabolism, it doesn't have too sound a basis, whereas within the concept of habit and personal comfort, it does. In the winter we get fatter simply because eating warm food and drinking brings a feeling of satisfaction and well-being, which in itself makes us feel more sluggish, lazier and less inclined to exercise. The two go hand in hand to create a bigger body. By the same token, the thought of losing weight – let alone just controlling it – through stringent eating and salad fare does not appeal at all. That, we tell ourselves, can wait till spring or summer; what is needed now is a good hot meal and a bit of flesh on the bones.

It's a reassuring argument, of course, and gets many of us off the guilt hook as regards over-indulgence. However, the fact is that we do not need extra fat to keep warm. The body has a remarkable thermostat system which is more than capable of adjusting to low temperatures without adverse effects (unless under extreme circumstances of dire cold, under-nourishment and immobility). The need for appetising, substantial food in cold weather is a psychological and not a physiological one. We like warmth, it makes us feel better, and if deprived of it through the elements we seek it through our food.

When it is cold, the body burns up more energy in order to maintain the biological equilibrium of temperature as well as to maintain the acid–alkaline balance in both the intra- and extra-cellular tissues. Body heat is thus retained or generated through a metabolic process and also through muscular exercise. Therefore, if you are not moving at all you need the 'inner flame' to provide warmth. When you eat, this is provided through the assimilation of food. Without food, the energy resources of stored fat are called upon to maintain body temperature. This, of course, makes you feel hungry – which would happen in warm weather just as much as in cold – but in the winter, the natural inclination and habit is to eat more in the misbelief that you need it to keep warm. In actual fact, you don't need the food – what you need (and get) is the continuance of a metabolic process that provides heat through the creation of energy. You don't need the feeling of satiety – comforting though it is to have it.

So fat is not necessary as a buffer against cold; thin people survive the winter just as well as the chubbier ones. Though certain fat is necessary – that which surrounds and protects the vital organs – the additional fat is there for an emergency, for when the body requires extra energy and food is not available. Most people think that fat exists as a inactive store-cupboard – and in fact this was the view of earlier medics too – but fat is really just as active an organ as any other. And it is actually a very large organ indeed, constituting from one fifth to one quarter of body weight in the normal person and half or more if you are grossly overweight. Its cells are extensively supplied with blood through a network of very small capillaries, and just like all other cells they have a constant shift in metabolism. Each cell represents a thermostat and has a pumping apparatus which draws fluids in and out through the cellular walls – a complex biochemical process that works for every millimetre of body tissue whether it be fat, vital organs or muscles. The maintenance of body heat relies on all cells, not just the fat ones. The real value of fat is not as an insulator but as a reserve source of heat-giving energy, and in that capacity the body needs only a thin layer.

Food intake, of course, as well as being a pleasant pastime, is the main provider of energy and its subsequent warmth. The body burns the foods through an intricate network of substances called enzymes, each one of which has a specific function genetically programmed in the chromosomes within the nuclei of every cell in the body. Oxygen is needed for this process. The carbohydrates (sugars, starches and the fibre in vegetables and fruits) and some fats are rapidly oxidised, some providing immediate energy (the sugars) and others a delayed source (the starches). Proteins – meat, fish, poultry, eggs – require the presence of some carbohydrate to be effectively assimilated and utilised, otherwise they have to draw on fat reserves to provide the burning fuel. This entire process produces energy, which equals heat – something only too obvious in hot weather when a hearty meal can make you sweat: this is not simply due to climatic heat, but also to that generated by the body during metabolism. In the cold weather, it is good to get that warm glow from food, but the fact remains that after doing the job of keeping the body at an even temperature, if the remaining energy is not used up in exercise or further combating the cold, it will get deposited as more fat.

Today, it is highly unlikely that you need constant protection from the cold. Hours spent indoors are cosily cushioned by central heating; hours spent outdoors are minimal. Unless you are out of doors and facing the elements all day, the whole idea of fat protection is a fallacy. And even then, you wouldn't need such fat protection if you were eating the kind of food that demands high-voltage body burning and thereby provides constant heat. Take the Eskimos, for example. They are not, in general, fat; under all that bulky clothing they are relatively lean. And yet they manage to keep warm in the worst of all climates. Why? Research has shown it is their diet; this consists mainly of fish, which requires the burning of stored resources for assimilation, and such a metabolic action produces a lot of heat.

The tendency is to eat more starchy foods in the cold weather as they make you feel full and contented, but, because of their delayed and extensive energy-providing factor, it is exactly these starches that easily turn into fat. No matter how worthy the wholegrains, if you eat a fair amount of them and are not very active, the residue is more likely to sit on your torso – rather than go sailing right through you as many people imagine. Fibre is vital and essential in the daily diet, but

3

it is easily obtainable in sufficient quantities in the vegetables and fruits.

So what is the answer in the winter months? If healthy eating is to be the rule – as it absolutely has to be – what sort of diet works for weight loss, and afterwards weight mainten-ance, and works for well-being and satisfaction as well? Most reducing diets are most off-putting in the cold when little food, or mostly raw food is very unappealing. Personal pam-pering is part of the winter syndrome. Yet in theory, winter should be the ideal time to lose weight. You need to burn up more energy if you are outside, but on the other hand you need to feel full and content as well. Feeling hungry and being cold just don't go together. Your metabolic rate is a significant factor too: those who burn up food quickly keep the heat up and the weight down, but ironically it is the lean ones who have this metabolism – and the overweight are left out in the cold, as it were, and with a slower burning rate. Exercise is cited as the way to step up metabolic rate, but the regimens suggested on many reducing diets (not less than half an hour brisk walking or jogging daily) are not to the liking – nor are they within the capacity – of many dieters.

Isn't there another way to trick the body into speeding up metabolism of food? Couldn't the cold be used to advantage – a way, through food, to give satisfaction and accelerate burn-ing power (without stimulating the desire to eat more) and to use up stored fat at the same time? Now there is: it's the new and revolutionary winter diet.

Chapter 2

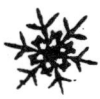

How to Lose Weight and Gain Health

It takes an original mind to come up with a palatable diet that works in the winter when everyone is inclined to eat and drink more. Over the past twenty years, a theory of how to lose weight and gain health within a limited time (eighteen days) has been worked out and put into action by Prof. Wolfgang G. Claren in practices in America, Italy and Germany and now in the Bad Dürrnberg clinic healthily tucked away in the Austrian Alps near Salzburg. It is a logical, scientific approach which has been empirically developed during the course of his day-to-day work in his speciality of geriatrics. Treating patients with disorders due to ageing, he found it was desirable for many to lose weight, positively helping the metabolic function at the same time.

Professor Claren has always been an advocate of the significant value of nutrition in preventive medicine. He was inveighing against the hazards of processed foods, sugar and salt long before such ideas became public property. He is, of course, all for natural, wholesome food, but his programme does not go to simplistic extremes. His is a worldly wise, realistic and knowledgeable medical attitude.

'We don't want to alter eating habits drastically, nor offer a rigid scheme. Our reducing plan should pose no problems, but through it we wish to make the reader think about his survival in a poisoned world and learn to best utilise what is at hand. We want to inspire you to think more before eating at home or in a restaurant – not to become a food faddist.'

The principle of the diet is this: beneficial use is made of the two different metabolic states – acid or alkaline – which occur during digestion of food. Certain foods produce a relatively acid background – mainly the animal, fish and bird sources – while others – mostly vegetables and fruits – produce an

5

alkaline liquid state. There are several vegetables, fruits and some fats which cause a balance of the acid–alkaline digestive juices, but they are not so relevant in the context of this particular diet. When the body is in an acid state, fat can be burned up faster, and when alkaline fluids are present, toxins are washed away as water is drawn from the cells, and the system is cleansed. Patients are put on three days of acid foods, then three days of alkaline, for a total of eighteen days. So for three days the body burns up fat, then for three days the body is purified. Pounds and inches are lost – and the metabolic system emerges much the better for it. That is putting it simply, too simply for Professor Claren, no doubt, but it seems the only way to present a very complex physiological process in understandable terms. The Professor refers to his regimen as 'The Swinging Diet' – appropriate indeed. This is the reasoning behind it . . .

The pathways of the digestive system are the crucial factors in the diet. The gut and digestive facilities show strictly separate pools for breaking up foods. There are juices specially prepared by a myriad of intestinal glands to break down proteins – and quite different ones to assimilate carbohydrates. In the case of carbohydrates, the first digestive juices ooze from underneath the tongue, continues in the stomach and finally the gut absorbs the broken-down sugar molecules. Proteins, on the other hand, are not attacked until they reach the acidity of the stomach.

'The management,' explains Professor Claren, 'has been designed throughout evolution and is similar in animals of all classes. Man, however, developed and refined his digestive system. Quick energy was provided in the upper anatomic parts of the digestive tract, an evolution which took place during the vegetarian times when man roamed the continents prior to his ability to make and use a tool. The transition from plant-eater to omnivorous animal meant many gradual alterations in the genetic programme – and today's man continues to carry the same instructions for vital enzymes, hormones, responses and cycles necessary for the digestion of food. We are geared to deal with a natural diet – of wild or domestic animals and unrefined fibrous vegetation; we are not geared to deal with today's over-refined, processed foods and the combinations of every type of food, though the body manages – much to its detriment at times. Our modern diet has unfurled over the last hundred years, a mere nothing compared to the millions of years of man's evolution, and it is unrealistic to expect the human organism to adjust and catch up.

'Of course, we do not want to return to the dark days of man's prehistory, nor do we wish to exercise any one of our ancestors' eating strategies. We merely want to use the digestive processes and the timetable of nature to trick our system, and so stimulate digestive juices into not only a cleansing action but also into regulating our stressed and artificially disjointed system into a more normal and natural gear.

'The three days acid and three days alkaline cycle matches the lifestyle pattern of predecessors, who fed on the carbohydrates (plant life) and then ate in abundance the proteins (from animals, fish, birds) when available. Indeed, it is generally beneficial not to change the digestive residual fluid within a span of twenty-four hours; this permits our digestive system to function in one gear only. But for the recuperative and reducing purposes of the Swinging Diet it has been found that the three-day pattern is the most desirable and effective.'

On the acid-residual days the diet is primarily animal protein, relieved with moderate servings of the vegetable carbohydrates which are considered balanced, neutral mixers. In nutrition circles, there is now a strong anti-animal-protein lobby which has greatly influenced people's eating habits. The hazards of protein depend on the type of protein (see pages 14–16) – and it seems odd and illogical that a food source which has been man's standby for nine-tenths of his evolution should suddenly be considered a dire threat to our health and survival. We need a certain amount of this protein (and some of its fats) together with the incorporated essential amino acids for building the body's nervous and arterial network and for providing physical strength. In the Swinging Diet, protein is used to its best advantage. The body becomes over acidified and because more oxygen is required for combustion, the burning capacity of the cells is increased and stored fat has to be mobilized to provide energy in the absence of adequate carbohydrate. This causes the production of ketobodies (acid chemical partitions); when these are produced to too great a degree – as in the case of a diabetic – they are a threat, but under the control of the three-day acid programme they are not harmful, and in addition they pave the way for the desired cellular washing (provided that the slimmer does not suffer from any metabolic disorder).

On the alkali-residual days the diet consists almost entirely of vegetables, with a few fruits (see pages 11-13). The change to the opposite digestive fluid activates a metabolic response which cleanses the body through intercellular exchanges of minerals and the washing away of toxins. The most significant minerals involved are sodium and potassium. Normal metabolism depends on the right balance between these two – and is the key to controlling blood pressure. We normally have too high a content of sodium (brought into the system through salt) and too little potassium through dietary deficiency.

'Even though the swing of this diet causes a temporary shock wave, this is both necessary and part of the plan, since it washes out the cellular fatigue caused by the over-presence of sodium and the undesired trace minerals which enter the cell during the acid-residual days. In this way we switch on the cellular pump and the inter-cellular liquids start shifting the sodium and potassium – and in doing so set the pace for an electric-like polarisation as from positive to negative. The "current" draws out certain trace minerals left from the acid state, leaving room for the entry of their counterparts from the alkaline residue. By using such a regulatory habitat we reduce water retention, clear out cellular slush and pollution.'

The diet consists of proteins, vegetables and fruits in their natural fibrous state, plus a few necessary fats. The cereal starches are not included despite the merits of wholegrains. This is because they pose several problems: during digestion the cereals require an acid milieu at one stage and an alkaline one at another. As a starch they cannot be combined with the protein on acid days otherwise they hamper the accelerated burning-up process. On alkaline days calories must be kept to a minimum – though they are not specifically counted in this diet – and in addition a more effective cleaning programme is carried out with just vegetables and fruits. There is no lack of fibre; plenty of this is available in the quantity of fresh vegetables consumed. Crucial to the success of the diet: minimum intake of salt.

The Key to the Diet: Alternating the Acid and Alkaline Foods

The three-day cycle swing from acid to alkaline body states lasts for eighteen days, which gives the system ample time to clear itself of the undesirable toxic matter and encourage greater inter-cellular activity – *and* it gives the body the opportunity to rid itself of an average of 5 lb (2.5 kilos) each week and the certainty of being inches thinner. These are the food allowances per day:

On the Acid Food Days

The hearty eating time, primarily consisting of substantial servings of fish, poultry or meat (a maximum of 200 grams for each meal) three times daily.
plus
salads selected from a wide variety of raw vegetables from the 'mixers' list of foods (see pages 11-13)
plus
the option of substituting one lightly cooked green vegetable
plus
the occasional fruit, but from a limited choice on the 'mixers' list
plus
the option of a small glass of dry white wine or dry cider with lunch and dinner
plus
the slimmer's aid of two egg-cups of cider vinegar (or any other fruit type) taken any time during the day
plus

9

any amount of herbal teas, three cups of coffee, half-and-half mixture of lemon (or orange) juice with mineral water, but no more than ½ pint of this mixture daily.

Blueprint for an acid day's fare:

Breakfast:	fish, mat or egg
	one raw vegetable
	tea or coffee
Lunch:	fish, meat or poultry
	large mixed salad
	glass white wine
Dinner:	fish, meat or poultry
	large mixed salad or one green cooked vegetable
	glass white wine
Any time:	herbal teas, two other cups of coffee, two egg-cups cider vinegar, the fruit juice (only if you need it)

On the Alkaline Food Days

A sparser time, but although the calorie intake should be watched (maximum of 800) it is unlikely to get too high because the bulk of the food allowed consists of the green vegetables which are full of fibre and are best for clearing out body slush. At one meal, it is recommended to take a large serving of a mixture of string beans and courgettes.
plus
fruit to start the day, a single choice or a large salad
plus
three other vegetable dishes, one raw combination from 'Mixers' list
plus
any amount of herbal teas, three cups coffee, half-and-half mixture of lemon (or orange) juice with mineral water, but no more than ½ pint daily.

Blueprint for an alkaline day's fare:

Breakfast: good helping of single fruit
                or combination salad
                tea or coffee

Lunch: steamed beans and courgettes
                or mixed salad

Dinner: vegetable soup
                cooked vegetable dish

Any time: herbal teas, three cups coffee, fruit juice

The Fundamental Rules

Although the diet swings from one food category to the other, there are basic principles that apply to both regimes and need to be closely observed.

✳ *use only fresh produce* and resist all temptation to substitute frozen, canned or packaged foods

✳ *give up sugar completely* which means puddings, cakes, jams, marmalades, sweets – and do not add it to anything

✳ *cereal starches are not permitted* during the Swinging Diet (though they can be returned to afterwards) and this includes even the healthy wholegrains and the breads made from them with the exception of the occasional use of brown rice as indicated in recipes. And *no* additions of flour or breadcrumbs.

✳ *keep within the range of listed foods* and be sure not to end up with a cross-combination meal if you switch any item on the detailed day-to-day plan given on pages 22 – 30

✳ *no extra snacks are allowed* between meals except for nibbling on the raw vegetables listed as 'Mixers'

✳ *be sure the cooking is right* (see pages 20 – 22) and note that small quantities of olive oil or butter have the seal of approval *(cont. on page 14)*

The Swinging Diet Foods

The following categorised lists clearly indicate which foods are permitted on the two regimens, and for the diet to have maximum effect they need to be strictly adhered to. The 'mixers' can move either way but are essentially additional items for interest or taste. The bulk of the diet has to come from the acid or alkaline selections.

ACID DAYS	MIXERS	ALKALINE DAYS
*cheese	*butter	artichokes
*dried pulses (peas, beans, lentils)	olive oil (cold pressed)	asparagus
	sunflower seed oil	aubergines (egg plant)
*dry cider	sesame seeds	*avocado
*dry white wine	yoghurt	beetroot
*eggs	yeast	broccoli
fish		cabbage (cooked)
game	Brussels sprouts	
meat	celery	courgettes (zucchini)
poultry	cabbage (raw)	kale
vinegar	carrots (raw or limited use in cooked dishes)	leeks
	chives	marrow
	cucumber	*parsnips
	dandelion leaves	*potatoes
	endive	*pumpkin
	fennel	spring greens
	garlic	string, or runner beans
	lettuce	*swedes
	mushrooms	*turnips
	mustard and cress	apples

ACID DAYS	MIXERS	ALKALINE DAYS
	onions	apricots
	parsley	*bananas
	peppers (green and red)	grapefruit
		melon
	spinach	papaya
	sprouted seeds	peaches
	← tomatoes (raw and cooked)	pears
	→ tomatoes (raw, but if cooked without skin and seeds)	pineapple
	watercress	
	blackcurrants	
	cherries	
	grapes	
	lemons	
	mandarins	
	mangoes	
	oranges	
	raspberries	
	strawberries	

*limited amounts
← for acid days only
→ for alkali days only

* *use salt sparingly,* otherwise you will retain water in the cells and impede good diet results
* *there's no need for vitamin supplements* because you are using fresh produce
* *ideal beverages are herbal teas* though it won't affect weight loss if regular tea or black coffee is drunk, and you can take a little milk with them if you like. Of course, it's a big *no* to all commercial soft drinks; and it's yes to mineral water and diluted lemon juice

Foods for Acid Days

The main life supporters are all foods which need an acid environment for food assimilation. These include the proteins such as meat, poultry, fish and eggs, the starch carbohydrates such as the grains and the cereals, also the dairy products of milk and cheese; then, in addition, the dried pulses (beans, peas, lentils) and the dreaded sugar. Of course, not all are suitable for this diet, not even the healthy and worthy wholegrains as explained before. These are the foods to concentrate on . . .

Fish: one of the most valuable foods, so eat as much of it as possible. If you happen to like fish a lot, substitute it for the meat or poultry on the diet plan. The protein content can be from 15 to 20 per cent, and fish also contains the desired balance of the essential amino acids. Fish supplies a complex of B vitamins and a healthy selection of vitamins and minerals. It contains varying amounts of fat, but of the important polyunsaturated genre. The fish low in fat are cod, haddock, plaice, sole, flounder, halibut, brill, sea bass and bream. The fattier ones are herrings, mackerel, sardines and salmon. Fresh-water fish, such as trout, pike, carp and perch, are also nutritionally good but marine fish have the added advantage of iodine absorption. Shel fish in particular provide significant amounts of iron and calcium; they are low in fat though high in cholesterol – lobsters have twice as much as meat, oysters even more.

Poultry and Game: chicken and turkey must be free range, then they are high in protein, low in fat, and have balanced amino acids and a good supply of vitamins and minerals. Battery-fed poultry has nothing to recommend it – it can be fat, water-logged and hormone-injected for rapid, profitable growth. Ducks and geese can be very fatty even if they were free roamers, so it's best to avoid them. Game, however, is just about the best and mostly uncontaminated protein source – rabbit, hare, venison – whilst wild birds (pheasant, grouse) are very nutritious, with lean meat providing excellent protein.

Meat: all meats provide high-quality protein with an ample supply of all the essential amino acids. They are rich in the B vitamins, especially B-1, B-2 and B-12; they contain iron, phosphorus, potassium, sodium and magnesium in appreciable amounts. Muscle meat (steaks, prime cut roasts) is a main source for protein replacement and its digestion eats up a lot of energy if the meat is lean and not overly cooked. Vitamins are retained if the steak is cooked no more than medium rare. However, the real value of meat depends on whether or not the animal has been injected with antibiotics or hormones in the interests of the greater value of greater weight. (British producers are still permitted to use hormones until 1989.) A certain amount of fat on meat is acceptable if it is naturally produced – and this is not detrimental to the diet. But the hazardous fat is the type which weaves its way through the flesh and fibres, giving the meat a 'marbled' look. Watch out for it. Of course, if the meat has a thick surface rim of fat, cut some away – but there's no need to get rid of every vestige. Beef, veal and lamb can all be eaten on the diet, but avoid pork including bacon, except for small amounts to spice up recipes. Organ meats should be taken in limitation: kidneys, preferably calf, use up considerable energy for digestion though they can contain a lot of sodium which is not so good. Liver is great value on the vitamin front but low in its capacity for digestive burning and use of body-stored calories. Absolutely and completely avoid all processed meat foods such as sausages, salami, luncheon meats, pâtés and pies – they all contain salt, sugar, colouring, chemical stabilizers and unhealthy consolidating components.

Eggs: fresh country eggs are best, and for this diet they should be hard-boiled, eaten cold without the yolk – and no more than two in the three-day acid cycle. Combined with tomatoes, they make a satisfying breakfast that really gets the metabolic burning going.

Cheese: use infrequently. Cheeses are fatteners as they contain a high percentage of fat and considerable salt. An occasional serving of fresh mozarella is all right, as is a sprinkling of Parmesan to enliven some dishes – but go easy. Even the much lauded cottage cheese has its drawbacks: it may be low in fat and salt, but the other mineral contents provide water-tagging molecules and so fluid retention can keep the inches on.

Dried Pulses: use infrequently, only when a hot soup is needed. Peas and beans provide fibre, protein and energy; they are also a good source of the B vitamins and some vitamin C. The dried seeds from pods are almost as rich in protein as fish and meat, but they don't give a big enough boost to the digestive metabolism, and are starchy.

Salad Vegetables: check the list of 'mixers' on the chart of diet foods and create salads from any combination (some suggestions are in the recipe section on pages 70-6). The most recommended are: watercress (a prime antioxidant), cucumber, fennel, tomatoes, green and red peppers. Only use onions, finely chopped, in small amounts to add flavour, as these are more valuable for the alkaline days. Garlic is superior for the acid regimen.

Cooked Vegetables: check the list of 'mixers' on the food chart. These may be used in recipes for composite dishes to make them tastier and also more appealing if meals for the family are required. Most worthy are: garlic, mushrooms, celery, tomatoes and peppers, while onions are a limited necessity for several dishes, though in this case they are considered neutralised because of cooking and being in combination with prime acid-residual foods. Try to avoid a cooked vegetable as an accompaniment to the main dish – it's not completely against the rules, but a serving of raw vegetables is far superior both for health and for diet results.

Fruits: an occasional treat, add only once during the three-day cycle and select only from those on the 'mixers' list. Lemons can be used in moderation for both cooking and for salads. Both the juice of lemons and orange can be diluted with an equal amount of mineral water and drunk between meals.

Condiments and other extras: butter can be used in reasonable amounts for cooking, as can cold-pressed olive oil for both cooking and as a salad dressing together with cider vinegar – this is very significant during acid days; use cider vinegar generously, but it must be of a fine quality, and *not* malt variety. Sunflower or sesame oils can substitute for olive oil. Garlic (a major antioxidant) can be employed generously. Yoghurt, the natural product, is fine in moderation. Powdered brewers' yeast should be tossed over dishes whenever possible – it has exceptional enzyme-enhancing value as well as containing all essential minerals and vitamins in a minute balanced measure. Parsley is the best and the most useful of garnishes – and it has the advantage of being an overall antioxidant.

Vinegar: cider and other fruit vinegars have the capacity to boost the burning-up process during metabolic digestion. The addition of two egg-cups of vinegar per acid day is highly recommended – some dieters may find it unpalatable to drink it neat, so if necessary dilute it with a little water.

Wine: for dieters who find it extremely difficult to abstain from alcohol – something that nearly all diets insist upon – the comfort here is that the Swinging Diet permits a small glass of dry white wine or dry cider with both lunch and dinner. Which wine is important: it must be very dry, fermented-through and containing not more than 1 per cent sugar and less than 20mg free sulphur. (Several wine producers and merchants now provide detailed lists of wine components – watch for them.) Very dry white wine will pull through the kidneys and stimulate the bowel.

Foods for Alkaline Days

This is limited to vegetables and fruits with an emphasis on their purgative qualities. At the Bad Dürrnberg Klinik and in the 18-day Swinging Diet concentration is on green string beans and courgettes, but there is considerable variety on the list of foods which also lend themselves to interesting dishes. Many vegetables can be made into simple soups, which are beneficial and more appealing on a cold day. Then there is the prime basic vegetable soup (recipe, page 64) which provides an abundance of potassium for the system.

Vegetables: these form 80 per cent of the alkaline diet and first choices should be the greens, which are high in vitamins and minerals – spinach, broccoli, cabbage and cauliflower are all valuable sources of vitamin C. Asparagus is rich in folic acid, one of the B vitamins that is often at a low level in a diet. Artichoke has a high potassium content. But to repeat, string beans and courgettes come first. The tuber and root vegetables should be used in moderation because although they are nutritionally good news they are high in calories. Onions should be used in combination with other vegetables for oven-baked dishes. Of the fruit vegetables, tomatoes are the most useful, but when cooked they need to be peeled and seeded, otherwise they become acid formers.

Salad Vegetables: these are taken from the 'mixers' list, but it is only necessary to have one large salad a day, which can also be a substitute for the ubiquitous string-bean-and-courgette combination should boredom set in (which is possible at times). Best choices: cucumber, celery, fennel, radishes, watercress and onions – plus raw tomatoes with skins.

Fruits: use all the fruits listed, concentrating on those in the alkaline list, but adding from the 'mixers' now and then for variety. Fruit can be taken singly or mixed together. Fruit is the breakfast meal for every alkaline day – and the only time of day it should be eaten. It is not recommended to combine fruit and vegetables in the same meal in this diet. Fruit provides a boost to the start of the day because of its energy-giving elements. The sugar carbohydrates (glucose, fructose or glactose) are converted mainly by the liver into glucose (blood-sugar) for energy. You can get all the sugar your body requires through fruit.

Condiments and other extras: use the minimum amount of butter and oil for the cooked dishes. For a salad dressing combine oil with lemon juice, no vinegar at all. Sunflower or sesame oils can substitute for olive oil as on acid days. Again use garlic, some yoghurt, brewers' yeast and parsley.

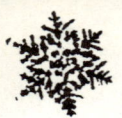

Chapter 3

The 18-day Swinging Diet

The basic formula couldn't be easier: it is simply a matter of making sure that only acid foods are eaten for three days, then only alkaline foods for three, with the convenient possibility of combining them with the 'mixer' foods. The specific diet is worked out to provide the most palatable regimen within the limits of biochemical control and nutrient necessities. However, it is not the only combination that works. The diet is individually flexible because there's a mass of food possibilities in both groups. You can work out your own plan and preferences if you follow the categorised food listings in the previous chapter.

The mapped-out diet has been geared to accommodate the realities of daily living. Breakfasts are quick, lunches are such that they could be found outside the home if necessary, and in addition to specific suggestions for dinner, recipes have been given for dishes that come strictly within the acid-or-alkaline rules but which also provide the basis of a family meal. The dieter can choose either. Just remember these salient facts:

✳ no breads any day

✳ on acid days you can eat heartily – up to 200 grams of fish, poultry or meat per meal – and it is preferable to take raw vegetables rather than cooked ones

✳ on alkaline days concentrate on vegetables rather than fruits and try to eat some string beans and courgettes every day

Cooking it Right

All the effort spent in planning the diet, selecting the best quality food and getting the acid – alkaline balance right can be to no avail if the cooking isn't right. If it is not right, nutrients can be destroyed and some elements actually altered. This may not involve very drastic changes, but it may be necessary to revise your thinking on some habitual methods of cooking. There are four cardinal rules:

✱ never fry in fat, although degrees of fats are allowed in the diet that doesn't mean in the frying pan

✱ meat, poultry and fish shold be grilled, boiled, roasted, poached or steamed – or cooked in a heavy skillet without the addition of any fat

✱ don't overcook anything, particularly vegetables

✱ keep an eagle eye on the salt, try to avoid it altogether, just a couple of grains if you must, but get used to using herbs as alternatives

Overcooking is probably the most common fault in British family cooking – even more prevalent than the tendency to fling everything in the frying pan. Unless a dish needs slow-cooking in the oven – as in a casserole – cooking time for all dishes should be short. Overdone food provides fewer of the essential nutrients, and value from food is particularly necessary when on a diet. It is only too easy to boil all the goodness out of vegetables; the vitamins and minerals are quickly drawn into the water and finally, of course, go down the drain. Ideally, vegetables should be steamed and they are often marvellously tasty when braised in the oven; if you can't kick the habit of boiling, then do so in the minimum amount of water and just to that point of crispness which requires some bite. Check out these methods:

Steaming: this can be done in a double-boiler, where water boils in the underneath section to heat the food above. But you can do it just as effectively by putting food in a colander or perforated rack over an ordinary pan of boiling water and cover it to accelerate cooking time. Leafy vegetables only take a few minutes, stalks and rots longer depending on maturity.

Fish also steams well.

Poaching: mostly for fish, but use a little water, lot of herbs and watch it carefully, because the more delicate varieties can disintegrate very quickly.

Boiling: always use the minimum amount of water except when cooking grains (rice and pasta) and the dried pulses. It is healthy to boil poultry and meats, but they need to be simmered slowly otherwise the flesh can become very tough.

Roasting: for meat, poultry and game. It is advisable to roast in the oven at a very high heat for the first 10 minutes to seal in the juices, then turn to a moderate heat for the required time. This helps prevent dryness and the need for additional fat (a no–no).

Grilling: a very healthy way to cook fish, steaks of meat and poultry. The food cooks in its own juices and if there is a lot of fat, this drips through the rack into the pan below – a far better place for it than your stomach.

Sautéing: adaptable for practically all foods – fish, poultry, meat and also many vegetables can be cooked in a heavy skillet. A little olive oil or butter may be necessary for a thin covering to prevent sticking or burning. This is quite different from frying – which involves a lot of fat. Sautéing is also the accepted way to bring out flavour: garlic, onions and several herbs thrive on it. Lower the heat after the first few minutes, over the pot and check constantly to prevent overcooking.

Stewing: this is casserole cooking, long and slow, and the classic way to prepare combination dishes of fish, meat or poultry with vegetables. However, it offers interesting alternatives for vegetable dishes with the added advantage of doing away with the need for water all of the time, and for oil or butter most of the time.

Foil-wrapping: a great method of retaining flavour and nutrients is to encase fish, meat or poultry in foil and allow it to cook-slowly in its own juices. No fat is added, just herbs and seasoning.

The Day-to-day Plan

Variety and personal preferences are very important in a diet, otherwise it is invariably abandoned. Here is the eighteen-day programme which clearly shows how palatable the Swinging Diet is, how understandable and direct to follow. In this form there have been good proven results. The alkaline days may appear a bit lean, but it's surprising how filling and tasty vegetables can be.

The diet doesn't have to be followed precisely, but whatever changes you make you *must* be sure you are substituting a comparable food. For example: fish, meat and poultry are interchangeable, so are the vegetables and fruits within their type and group, though the quantity of tubers should be limited. Also eggs cannot be used any way other than hardboiled. Don't add cheese (even a sprinkling) unless indicated. If you feel you need it, you may have a glass of dry white wine or cider with lunch and dinner but *only* on the acid days and providing it's the right type (see page 17). Adding a couple of egg-cups of cider or fruit vinegar on acid days is also a help to slimming. The recipes for ★ dishes are in Chapter 4, and there are many alternatives to try, plus a section of ideas for the 'mixer' salads. Use the eye to judge quantities unless they are stated — average portions of the prepared dishes and vegetables, a bowl of soup, a large bowl of salad.

N.B. ✳ Refer to the acid and alkaline food lists on pages 11–12 in order to select vegetables and fruits when not specified here.

✳ Salads on both the acid and alkaline days are to be made up from the selection of 'mixer' vegetables unless otherwise stated.

✳ If in-between snacks are found to be an absolute necessity, nibble on vegetables from the 'mixer' list.

✳ herbal teas are preferable to coffee either taken after meals or between them; lemon or orange juice diluted with an equal amount of mineral water may also be drunk between meals.

DAY 1   ACID

Breakfast	Lunch	Dinner
2 cold hard-boiled eggs, whites only 2 raw tomatoes	steak, medium/rare up to 200g salad selected from 'mixers'	grilled, baked or poached fish up to 200g 2 grilled tomatoes watercress *or* ★Baked Fish with Olives salad selected from 'mixers'

DAY 2   ACID

poached, baked or grilled fish up to 200g 2 raw tomatoes	grilled kidneys *or* steak medium/rare up to 200g salad selected from 'mixers'	braised or grilled chicken breasts up to 200g *or* ★Boiled Chicken both with salad selected from 'mixers'

DAY 3   ACID

grilled liver (2 slices) 2 raw tomatoes	grilled, baked or poached fish up to 200g salad selected from 'mixers'	steak medium/rare up to 200g *or* ★Alpine Stew both with either spinach or cabbage

DAY 4   ALKALI

mixed fruit salad selected from choice on alkaline list	steamed or boiled string beans and courgettes *or* large vegetable salad selected from both alkaline and 'mixer' lists	*Basic Vegetable Soup (large bowl)

DAY 5   ALKALI

single fruit: 1 grapefruit *or* 2 slices melon *or* 2 slices pineapple *or* 2 apples	steamed or boiled string beans and courgettes *or* large vegetable salad selected from both alkaline and 'mixer' lists	steamed brocolli and cauliflower *or* *Leek and Tomato Casserole

DAY 6   ALKALI

mixed fruit salad from choice on both alkaline and 'mixer' lists	steamed or boiled string beans and courgettes *or* large vegetable salad selected from both alkaline and 'mixer' lists	large portion of any cooked green vegetable together with onions *or* *Stuffed Aubergines

DAY 7   ACID

2 cold hard–boiled eggs, whites only 2 raw tomatoes	steak medium/rare up to 200g salad selected from 'mixers'	grilled, baked or poached fish up to 200g 2 raw tomatoes green peppers and watercress *or* ★Fish Soup

DAY 8   ACID

grilled liver (2 slices) *or* grilled kidneys 2 raw tomatoes	grilled, baked or poached fish up to 200g salad selected from 'mixers'	4 slices roast chicken *or* ★Turkey Casserole both with salad selected from 'mixers'

DAY 9   ACID

poached or grilled fish up to 200g 2 grilled tomatoes	4 slices hot or cold roast chicken or turkey salad selected from 'mixers'	steak medium/rare up to 200g salad selected from 'mixers' *or* ★Veal with Mushrooms cooked spinach *or* salad selected from 'mixers'

DAY 10   ALKALI

mixed fruit salad selected from choice on alkaline list	steamed or boiled string beans and courgettes *or* large vegetable salad selected from both alkaline and 'mixer' lists	large portion of any cooked green vegetable with onions *or* ★Carrot and Orange Soup and ★1 Jacket Potato with any filling listed in the recipe

DAY 11   ALKALI

single fruit: 1 grapefruit *or* 2 slices melon *or* 2 slices pineapple *or* 2 apples	steamed or boiled string beans and courgettes *or* large vegetable salad selected from both alkaline and 'mixer' lists	steamed broccoli and cauliflower *or* ★Baked Aubergines

DAY 12   ALKALI

mixed fruit salad from choice on both alkaline and 'mixer' lists	steamed or boiled string beans and courgettes *or* large vegetable salad selected from both alkaline and 'mixer' lists	★Basic Vegetable Soup (large bowl)

DAY 13   ACID

grilled liver or kidney	steak medium/rare up to 200g	grilled, baked or poached fish up to 200g
2 grilled tomatoes	salad selected from 'mixers'	*or* ★Cod Kebab
		both with salad selected from 'mixers'

DAY 14   ACID

2 cold hard–boiled eggs, whites only	grilled, baked or poached fish up to 200g	braised or grilled chicken breasts up to 200g
2 raw tomatoes	salad selected from 'mixers'	*or* ★Chicken Winter Stew
		both with salad selected from 'mixers'

DAY 15   ACID

poached or grilled fish up to 200g	4 slices of hot or cold roast chicken, turkey or veal	steak medium/rare up to 200g
2 grilled tomatoes	salad selected from 'mixers'	*or* ★Sautéd Beef with Yoghurt
		both with salad selected from 'mixers' or spinach or Brussels sprouts

DAY 16 ALKALI

mixed fruit salad selected from choice on alkaline list	steamed or boiled string beans and courgettes *or* large vegetable salad selected from both alkaline and 'mixer' lists	Mixed green vegetables steamed with onions *or* ★Hot Cucumber Soup and ★Lemon Cauliflower

DAY 17 ALKALI

single fruit: 1 grapefruit *or* 2 slices melon *or* 2 slices pineapple *or* 2 apples	★Basic Vegetable Soup	★Ratatouille (large helping)

DAY 18 ALKALI

mixed fruit salad from choice on both alkaline and 'mixer' lists	steamed or boiled string beans and courgettes *or* large vegetable salad selected from both alkaline and 'mixer' lists	steamed broccoli and cauliflower *or* ★Stuffed Peppers

Healthy Eating After the 18-day Diet

The prime purpose of the Swinging Diet is, of course, to lose pounds and inches, but through it the dieter can also acquire a new awareness of the biochemical nature of certain foods and their contributory value to general health. The fundamentals of the diet can successfully be incorporated into the average daily eating plan. The acid – alkaline balance continues to be significant, but in a different way: 80 per cent of food should be alkaline and 20 per cent acid, but these foods can now be eaten on the same day and at the same meal. However, Professor Claren points out that a healthy move is to have an all-alkaline meal every few days to help clean out the system. Grains – cereals, bread, rice, pasta – can now be added, but because these are starches, they should be eaten in moderation; for health, they should preferably be in their wholegrain, unrefined state. The grains are acid-forming foods. The most important thing to watch is the intake of acid foods, as most people's eating habits involve a much higher proportion than the ideal of 20 per cent. This means cutting down on meat, poultry, fish, eggs and cereals – and increasing quantities of vegetables, salads and fruits. The general rules to follow are:

* cut convenience and processed foods to a minimum, cut them out entirely if possible

* aim for fresh produce

* include a wide variety of foods in your diet

* replace refined flours and cereals with wholegrains

* eat few sweet foods and replace white sugar with unrefined varieties or honey

* eat a lot of fibre foods with emphasis on the vegetables and fruits

* make an effort to eat some raw food every day

* watch fat intake

* use the same cooking rules as for the diet

* use a minimum amount of salt
* keep alcohol at a moderate level

A Daily Guide

When and what you eat depends on individual lifestyle, but most people usually have a quick breakfast or give it a miss (you shouldn't), lunch has invariably to be geared to possibilities at the work place, while the evening meal can be planned at home and under nutritional control. Here's a practical way to balance the 80 per cent acid and 20 per cent alkaline food.

Breakfast: wholegrains and fresh fruit are the best choices: porridge, muesli, a slice of bread, fresh fruit or dried fruits soaked overnight; yoghurt, butter for the bread, some honey or home-made preserves – coffee or tea.

Lunch: cncentrate on vegetables and salads – even when eating in a canteen or restaurant there is now normally a selection of vegetables and salads. Pasta or rice dishes are also a good choice, together with a salad; fruit for dessert. Sandwiches are healthy only if you use wholegrain bread; use lots of salad fillings (avoid processed meats) tinned tuna fish, salmon and sardines are fine, so are the low-fat cheeses.

Dinner: the most convenient meal for the acid-related proteins of meat, poultry or fish as you can control the quality of both produce and cooking. It is healthier to eat more fish, less meat. Balance the protein with two or three fresh vegetables or salads. In the winter months, add a nourishing vegetable soup. Select fresh fruit for dessert, reserving cheese for occasional treats only.

It is the refined sugars and flours that are the villains of nutrition and both should be cut down to a minimum – the occasional cake, chocolate, biscuit, sauce or sweet is not going to harm, but regular daily consumption is clearly a health hazard. Fat intake has to be watched too. This means avoiding fried foods, using butter or margarine in small amounts, limiting eggs to three a week, consuming only a little cheese. Olive oil is the healthiest medium for cooking and for salad dressings.

Chapter 4

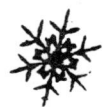

Recipes for the Acid-or-Alkaline Way of Dieting

On the following pages is a selection of recipes which indicate the type of appealing and appetising dishes which can be achieved working within the confines of the acid and alkaline food categories – and the diet. Some of them have been included in the specific 18-day Swinging Diet, but there are many additions and substitutions you can make as you choose. They are hearty, healthy ideas for the whole family to enjoy (recipes are planned to serve four) and offer a acceptable variety for the dieter.

The excellence of any dish depends on the quality of the ingredients: fresh produce is a cardinal rule. Most of the recipes are quick and easy, and because it is essential to cut down on salt (the smallest pinch only is permitted), liberal use is made of herbs. Through herbs you can give special flavour to basic dishes. They should be used according to your personal palate; there's no need to have a vast array – start with dill, marjoram, rosemary, sage, tarragon and thyme. And always have fresh parsley, mint and basil at hand in the kitchen – for health, for taste and for looks as a garnish. The acid-day recipes are for fish, meat and poultry, as well as winter soups and sauces. The alkaline-day recipes are for substantial vegetable dishes, soups and sauces. There are also suggestions for 'mixer salads' which can be eaten with either regimen. Note that any dry white wine you may use in some of the acid day recipes count as part of your daily allowance.

Recipes For Acid Days: Fish

Classic Fish Fillets
8 fish fillets (preferably white fish)
2 bay leaves
½ cup dry white wine (or dry cider)
25g (1 oz) butter
2 tablespoons chopped parsley or chives
sea salt and pepper

Roll the fillets, secure with toothpicks and place in a lightly oiled casserole. Season with a little salt and some freshly ground pepper. Dab with butter, pour over the wine or cider, add the bay leaves and cook for 30 to 45 minutes in a moderate oven (350°F, 175°C, gas 4). Garnish with parsley or chives.

Cod Kebab
350g (12 oz) cod
8 – 12 small onions
2 green peppers
4 bay leaves
a little olive oil
salt, freshly ground pepper
handful of chopped parsley

Cut the fish into substantial cubes; peel onions; seed and remove pith from green peppers and cut into 5-cm (2-inch) pieces. Cook the fish, peppers and onions in lightly salted boiling water for 5 minutes. Drain. Arrange fish, onions and peppers on skewers, threading a bay leaf onto each. Sprinkle with salt and freshly ground pepper; lightly brush with olive oil. Grill for about 8 to 10 minutes. Before serving, garnish with parsley.

Baked Fish with Olives

1 or 2 plump whole fish such as mullet, mackerel, bream, brill, bass
3 medium onions
4 medium tomatoes
½ cup chopped parsley
10 stoned black olives
½ cup dry white wine (or dry cider)
sea salt, freshly ground pepper

Peel and slice the onions, chop the tomatoes after first removing skin and seeds. Arrange half of each in a layer on the bottom of a baking dish. Sprinkle on a little salt, freshly ground pepper and the chopped parsley. Place the cleaned fish on this bed. Cover with another layer of onions and tomatoes interspersed with olives, cut in half. Pour the wine over the layers. Cover with foil and bake in a moderate oven (350°F, 175°C, gas 4) for 30 to 45 minutes or until the fish is tender. Garnish with chopped parsley.

Poached Trout

4 trout
4 cups water
¼ cup cider vinegar
2 onions, sliced
2 carrots, chopped
8 peppercorns
1 bay leaf
½ teaspoon thyme
handful of chopped parsley
sea salt

Prepare the poaching liquid by simmering the water, cider vinegar, onions, carrots, bay leaf, thyme, salt and peppercorns for about an hour. Put the trout, previously headed, in another pan, brush with a little additional cider vinegar. Pour the prepared stock over the fish. Reduce the heat and gently poach for 15 minutes. Serve generously sprinkled with parsley.

Marinated Trout

4 small trout
15 ml (1 tablespoon) olive oil
½ cup dry white wine (or dry cider)
15 ml (1 tablespoon) honey
4 shallots, chopped
1 teaspoon cumin
salt and pepper
1 tablespoon chopped chives
handful of chopped parsley
olive oil for brushing

Clean the trout. Make a marinade from the oil, wine, honey, shallots, cumin, salt and pepper. Immerse the fish and let them marinate for 1 to 2 hours. Remove the fish and brush with olive oil. Wrap in foil, place on a flat dish and bake in a moderate oven (350°F, 175°C, gas 4) for about ½ hour or until the fish is cooked through. Serve garnished with finely chopped chives and parsley.

Fish Casserole

680 g (1½ lb) white fish – cod, haddock or plaice
450 g (1 lb) tin Italian plum tomatoes
125 g (4 oz) button mushrooms
10 ml (2 teaspoons) Worcestershire sauce
sea salt, freshly ground pepper
2 tablespoons grated Parmesan cheese (optional, and not for strict dieters)

Clean and flake the fish and put in the bottom of a casserole dish. Stir the Worcestershire sauce into the tomatoes and their liquid, season with a little salt and pepper. Pour over the fish and finally top with mushrooms, finely sliced. Bake in a moderate oven (350°F, 175°C, gas 4) for 20 to 30 minutes. Serve with a sprinkling of Parmesan cheese if desired.

Steamed Mussels in Wine
3 litres (6 pints) mussels
1 medium onion
30 ml (2 tablespoons) olive oil
2 garlic cloves
½ cup water
½ cup dry white wine (or dry cider)
handful of chopped parsley
freshly ground pepper

Clean and scrape the mussels. Warm the oil in a wide frying pan. Put in the mussels together with the chopped garlic and onion. Pour over the wine and water. Cover and bring to the boil, cooking over a high heat for about 5 minutes or until the mussels open. Discard any mussels that have not opened. Drain and reserve the liquid, season with pepper (the mussels usually provide enough of their own salt) and stir in the chopped parsley. Pour the liquid over the mussels.

Continental Prawns
450 g (1 lb) prawns ★
1 medium onion
1 garlic clove
1 green pepper
4 medium tomatoes
15 ml (1 tablespoon) olive oil
1 teaspoon dried oregano
¼ cup dry white wine (or dry cider)
sea salt, freshly ground pepper
handful of chopped parsley

Chop tomatoes into chunks, retaining both skins and seeds. Peel and finely cut up the onion. Seed and remove pith of green pepper, then chop into pieces. Heat the olive oil in a deep pan, add the garlic (crushed or finely chopped), cook for a minute, add the onion and green pepper and cook for a

★ *It is all right to use frozen prawns.*

further 5 minutes. Put in the tomatoes and pour in the white wine; season with a little salt, pepper and oregano. Cover the pan, reduce heat and simmer for 10 to 15 minutes. Add the peeled prawns and continue to cook at the same heat for 5 minutes. Sprinkle with parsley to serve.

Fish Soup

900 g (2 lb) mixed fresh fish
handful of shelled prawns (frozen permitted)
bits of lobster (if you can find them, but not essential)
3 cloves garlic (peeled only)
1 medium onion, peeled and chopped
2 medium tomatoes, chopped
½ cup olive oil
½ cup water
¼ cup dry white wine (or dry cider)
sprig of fresh thyme (or 1 teaspoon dried)
sprig of fennel (optional, only if available)
2 bay leaves
a pinch of saffron (optional)
sea salt, freshly ground pepper
handful of chopped parsley

Cut all the fish into small pieces. Heat the oil in a large deep pot, cook the onion for a few minutes (stew not fry it) then add the garlic, parsley and tomatoes. Season with a little salt and pepper. Pop in the herbs of thyme, fennel and bay leaves. A pinch of saffron gives a more spicy flavour, but this is optional. Pour in the wine and water. Stir well. Bring to the boil and immediately lower the heat, allowing the broth to simmer for about 20 minutes. If it looks too thick, simply add some hot water. Take out the bay leaves. Add the mixed fresh fish (remove any skin), simmer for 5 to 8 minutes, now add any lobster pieces, continue to simmer for 5 minutes and finally add the prawns which need only a further 2 or 3 minutes. Check all fish is tender. Garnish with chopped parsley.

Recipes For Acid Days: Poultry

Boiled Chicken

1 fresh, fee-range chicken
1 medium onion, quartered
1 stick celery, whole
1 carrot, peeled
1 teaspoon thyme
1 bay leaf
1 blade mace (optional)
8 peppercorns
½ lemon
handful of parsley
sea salt

It is not necessary to get a boiling chicken, a fresh 'roasting' chicken can be boiled; in fact it is quicker to cook and often tenderer. A boiling fowl is often fatter too – something to be avoided. Remove any excess fat on the chicken. Put in a very deep pot together with all vegetables and herbs. Grate the ½ lemon and juice it. Add to the chicken and then season with just a little sea salt; drop in the peppercorns. Pour in enough water to almost cover the chicken. Bring to the boil, lower heat and simmer gently for about an hour or until the chicken is tender. Be sure to skim off any fat. Drain the chicken and reserve the stock. Serve garnished with parsley.

Grilled Rosemary Chicken

1 fresh, free-range chicken
30 ml (2 tablespoons) olive oil
2 teaspoons finely crushed rosemary
freshly ground pepper
sea salt

Remove any obvious excess fat from the chicken. Cut lengthwise into two pieces and flatten. Mix together the oil, rosemary, a little salt, freshly ground pepper. Rub this into the skin of the chicken. Grill under a fairly fast heat, turning the chicken several times to ensure even browning, and basting with a little more oil if necessary to prevent dryness. The chicken should cook in about 20 minutes.

Chicken Winter Stew

1 fresh, free-range chicken
45 ml (3 tablespoons) olive oil
2 cloves garlic
1 medium onion
1 green pepper
1 red pepper
125 g (4 oz) mushrooms (optional)
450 g (1 lb) can Italian plum tomatoes
½ cup water
sea salt, freshly ground pepper
handful of freshly chopped parsley

Cut the chicken into pieces (the butcher will do this). Heat the olive oil in a deep pan and slowly cook the chopped garlic and onion for a few minutes. Add the chicken and brown on all sides. Remove the pith and seeds from the peppers, cut into slices and add to the pan. Pour in the tomatoes and add the mushrooms; season with a little salt and freshly ground pepper. Add the water, stir well. Cover and cook slowly for about 1 hour or until the chicken is tender. Serve garnished with freshly chopped parsley.

Coq au Vin

1 chicken
2 medium onions
2 garlic cloves
1 bay leaf
½ litre (1 pint) red wine
25 g (1 oz) butter
225 g (8 oz) button mushrooms
sea salt
freshly ground pepper

Chop the chicken into pieces (ask the butcher to do this). Melt the butter in a skillet; add the chicken and brown evenly on all sides. Transfer to a casserole dish. Cook the chopped onion and garlic in the residue fat then drain them on kitchen paper. Add onion and garlic to the chicken, toss in the bay leaf, pour over the wine and season with a little salt and pepper. Cook in a hot oven (425°F, 220°C, gas 5) for about 1 to 1½ hours. Wash and slice the mushrooms; add to the casserole and cook for a further 15 minutes.

Turkey Casserole

450 g (1 lb) turkey pieces
2 cloves garlic
25 g (1 oz) butter
1 medium onion
2 carrots
1 celery stick
1 teaspoon dried thyme
2 bay leaves
1 thick slice bacon
2 cups chicken stock
300 ml (½ pint) dry white wine (or dry cider)
½ lemon
sea salt
freshly ground pepper

Melt the butter in a deep pan and gently cook the sliced onion; add the turkey pieces and brown on all sides. Peel the carrots and slice into long strips; add to the pan together with whole, peeled garlic cloves and chopped celery. Put in the slice of bacon (uncut), thyme and bay leaves; pour over the white wine. Cook over a low heat for about 10 to 15 minutes, moving the ingredients around from time to time to see nothing gets scorched. Now add the chicken stock, season with a little salt and ample freshly ground pepper. Cover and simmer on a very low heat for about 1½ hours or until the turkey is tender. Lift out the turkey pieces and keep them warm; remove the bay leaves; put the rest of the stock and vegetables through a blender (first cutting the bacon into small pieces). Add the grated rind and juice of ½ lemon. Pour the sauce over the turkey pieces.

Recipes for Acid Days: Meat

Veal with Mushrooms

8 thick slices of veal
25 g (1 oz) butter
juice of ½ lemon
125 g (4 oz) button mushrooms
½ cup dry white wine (or dry cider)
sea salt
freshly ground pepper

Beat the veal slices so they are flat. Season with pepper and
lemon juice and a little salt. Clean and slice the mushrooms
and cover with rest of lemon juice. Allow to marinate for a
few minutes. Meanwhile melt the butter and when really hot
drop in pieces of veal and quickly brown them on both sides.
Add mushrooms, pour over the wine and after letting it
bubble for a minute, turn down the heat and simmer for a
couple of minutes.

Veal (or Beef) Kebabs

900 g (2 lb) lean veal (or beef)
450 g (1 lb) button mushrooms
2 green peppers
45 ml to 60 ml (3 to 4 tablespoons) olive oil
2 garlic cloves
¼ cup soy sauce
salt

Cut the veal (or beef) into 2-cm (1-inch) squares. Make a
marinade with the oil, little salt, crushed garlic cloves and soy
sauce. Stir well and marinate the meat in the refrigerator for
about 5 hours. Seed the peppers, remove the pith and cut into
substantial pieces. Clean the mushrooms but don't cut unless
very large. On a skewer alternate veal and mushrooms and
peppers. Grill until brown and tender (about 10 to 15
minutes).

Sautéd Beef with Yoghurt Sauce

450 g (1 lb) lean beef steak
2 medium onions
125 g (4 oz) button mushrooms
50 g (2 oz) butter or margarine
a little olive oil
sea salt
freshly ground pepper
1 cup natural yoghurt
handful of chopped parsley

Remove any fat from the meat and cut into thin strips. Peel
and slice the onions; clean and slice the mushrooms. Melt the
butter or margarine in a large pan and first fry the onions until
golden, then add the mushrooms and cook for only a couple of
minutes. In another pan, heat the olive oil over a high flame,
drop in the beef strips and quickly sauté so they are brown on
the outside but still slightly pink within. Put on kitchen paper
to drain off any excess oil, then add to the onions and mushrooms. Stir well together (with a wooden spoon) and season
with a little salt and pepper, continuing to cook over a low
flame for about 2 minutes. Gradually stir in the yoghurt,
keeping the heat low so the dish never gets above simmering
point. At the last minute, sprinkle with chopped parsley.

Alpine Stew

1-1½ kilos (2-3 lb) beef for boiling (brisket)
4 medium-sized onions
2 garlic cloves
3 carrots
1 small cabbage
6 peppercorns
1 bay leaf
1 teaspoon dried thyme
1 tablespoon chopped parsley
2 sticks celery
sea salt

Remove any fatty areas from the beef, roll and tie with string, sprinkle with a little salt and put in a very deep pot and cover with cold water. Peel the garlic cloves and add them whole; cut the celery into 2-cm (1-inch) pieces and put in the pot together with the peppercorns, bay leaf, thyme and parsley. Bring to the boil, skimming off any fat or scum that rises to the surface. Cover, reduce heat and simmer ently for about 2 hours. Peel and chop the onions and carrots; add to the pot and simmer for a further hour. Cut the cabbage into small segments, add to the stew and cook for another 20 minutes. The beef must be very tender and the vegetables not over-cooked. The beef should be drained and the vegetables placed around it for serving.

Mixed Boiled Meats

900 g (2 lb) fresh beef tongue
450 g (1 lb) cotechino sausage (or any uncooked garlic sausage)
900 g (2 lb) boneless joint of beef (silverside, topside)
1 fresh, free-range chicken
4 onions
8 carrots
4 sticks celery
2 bay leaves
8 peppercorns
sea salt
bunch of fresh parsley

This is, of course, much more than a dish for four, however it can be reheated and also served cold. It is great for a dinner party and no one will ever guess you are following a diet. First cook the tongue; cover with cold water, bring to the boil and then simmer for about 3 hours or until tender. Drain, skin and remove the fat and gristle at the base. Prick the sausage (to prevent splitting), put in a pan and cover with cold water. Bring to the boil, then simmer for about 40 minutes. In a very large pan (if you haven't got a big one, you will have to cook the meats separately) put the beef (rolled and tied), the quartered onions, peeled whole carrots, celery sticks, bay leaves, parsley sprigs and peppercorns; cover with cold water, add a little salt, bring to the boil, skim off any foam, then simmer for 90 minutes. Add the chicken, continue simmering for 20 minutes. Add the tongue and sausage. Simmer together for a further ½ hour or until all the meats are tender. During cooking remove any fat or scum that appears on the surface. Strain the meats (the liquid can be reserved as a stock); skin the sausage. Slice the meats and sausage, carve the chicken and serve hot on a platter, accompanied by Green Sauce (see recipe, page 51).

Marinated Boned Lamb
a good leg of lamb – 1½-2 kilos (3-4 lb) boned
2 medium onions
1 clove garlic
75 ml (5 tablespoons) olive oil
30 ml (2 tablespoons) wine or cider vinegar
5 ml (1 teaspoon) sea salt
1 teaspoon peppercorns
½ teaspoon oregano
1 bay leaf

Crush the garlic and break up the bay leaf into small pieces. Peel and finely chop the onions. Combine all ingredients to make the marinade and stir with a wooden spoon. Soak meat overnight in the refrigerator. Next day, drain and put leg, fat side up, on a rack in a shallow pan. Brush meat with marinade. Roast for 10 minutes in a hot oven (450°F, 250°C, gas 8) – the surface should be golden brown; then reduce heat and cook in a slower oven (300°F, 150°C, gas 3) for 2 to 2½ hours.

Venetian Calf's Liver
450 g (1 lb) calf's liver
4 medium onions
30 ml (2 tablespoons) olive oil
sea salt
freshly ground pepper
handful of chopped parsley
glass red wine (optional)

Slice the onions very finely and cut the liver into the very thinnest slices. Warm the oil and put in the onions which should be sautéd slowly until golden brown. Add a little salt. Now turn up the heat a little and drop in the liver slices. These should be cooked very fast – a mere minute for each side. Add the wine (if you like), season with pepper and serve sprinkled with chopped parsley.

Lamb's Liver with Basil

1 large (or 2 small) lamb's liver
2 slices lean bacon
25 g (1 oz) butter
½ cup red wine (optional)
4 tablespoons chopped basil
1 cup chicken stock (permissible to make from a cube)
sea salt
freshly ground pepper

Wash and finely slice the liver. Cut the bacon into pieces and fry it in its own fat. In another pan, heat the butter and when hot sauté the liver very quickly – it should be brown on the outside and pink within, and this is only possible when cooking is hot and fast. Add the chopped basil, a little salt and freshly ground pepper, pour over the wine (optional), then the chicken stock. Simmer for a few minutes only. Serve with a sprinkling of crisp, crushed bacon and aditional freshly chopped basil.

Kidneys with Parsley and Wine

8 kidney segments (calves' are the best)
25 g (1 oz) butter
1 cup red wine
1 small onion
½ cup chopped parsley
freshly ground pepper

Clean the kidneys and put them into hot salted water for 5 minutes. Drain and then marinate them for 2 hours in half of the wine, which has previously been warmed. Finely chop the onion and cook in the melted butter until golden. Cut the kidneys into slices, add to the onion. Cook slowly for about 20 minutes, gradually adding the rest of the wine. During the last few minutes sprinkle with chopped parsley and a little freshly ground pepper.

Kidneys with Mushrooms

8 lamb kidney segments
25 g (1 oz) butter
125 g (4 oz) mushrooms
10 very small onions
900 g (1 lb) can Italian plum tomatoes
1 bay leaf
sea salt
freshly ground pepper
handful of chopped parsley

Plunge the kidneys into boiling water for a minute; skin and core them, cut into slices. Melt the butter, quickly brown the kidneys on both sides, add mushrooms (cleaned and sliced) then the small whole onions (peeled). Stir for a minute. Add the entire contents of the can of tomatoes, drop in the bay leaf, season with very little salt and a generous amount of freshly ground pepper. Lower the heat, cover and simmer for 15 minutes until tender. Remove bay leaf. When serving, garnish with chopped parsley.

Recipes For Acid Days: Soups

Winter Bean Soup

1 cup dried white beans
1 clove garlic
olive oil
bunch of parsley
sea salt
freshly ground pepper

Soak the beans overnight, drain. Put in a pan and generously cover with water. Boil slowly until tender – this may take 2 to 3 hours and it may be necessary to skim off froth from time to time. Put through a sieve or colander, but retain the liquid. Return beans to the pan with as much of the reserved liquid as is necessary to make a good thick bean soup. Now add a little salt and pepper. In another pan, heat a little olive oil and add the clove of garlic, finely chopped. When it is just about to turn colour (never let it brown or burn) add a handful of chopped parsley. Take immediately from the heat. Add this to the soup just before serving.

Mixed Bean Soup

½ cup dried haricot beans
½ cup dried black-eyed peas
½ cup dried kidney beans
¼ cup split red lentils
1 clove garlic
1 large carrot
1 large onion
1 celery stick
15 ml (1 tablespoon) olive oil
chopped parsley
sea salt
freshly ground pepper

Soak the haricot beans, black-eyed peas and kidney beans overnight. Drain. Put all the beans in a large pot together with peeled garlic clove, whole peeled carrot, whole peeled onion and the cleaned celery stick. Cover with a lot of water and boil gently for about 1½ hours. Add the lentils and boil for a further 45 minutes. Keep checking to see if there is enough water. Remove the garlic, carrot, onion and celery stick. Season with sea salt and pepper. Before serving stir in the olive oil and garnish with chopped parsley.

Pea Soup with Tarragon

225 g (8 oz) dried peas
4 cups water
2 tablespoons chopped fresh tarragon (or 1 tablespoon dried)
natural yogurt
sea salt
freshly ground pepper

Soak the peas for about an hour then boil until soft. Add the tarragon and simmer for a further 10 minutes. Season to taste. Put through the blender and stir in the yogurt before serving.

Recipes For Acid Days: Sauces

Classic Oil and Vinegar Dressing
(for salads, raw or cold cooked vegetables)
1 part wine or cider vinegar
3 parts dark green olive oil
a little salt
freshly ground pepper

The better the ingredients, the better the dressing – that is why it is preferable to use the very best dark green virgin olive oil, vegetable oils just don't taste the same. The ingredients need to be well stirred or shaken into a smooth mix. There are many alternative additions: a crushed garlic clove, a little Dijon or English mustard, freshly chopped herbs such as chives, parsley or basil – these added at the very last minute before serving.

Basic Yoghurt Sauce
(very versatile, for salads, raw vegetables, fish, meat and chicken dishes)
½ cup natural yogurt
¼ cup cider vinegar
8 ml (½ tablespoon) green olive oil
freshly ground pepper
a few grains of salt

Simply mix all ingredients together until thoroughly blended. While this simple sauce is great for salads, it is also the basis for a variety of delicious tastes. These are some possibilities: add 1 clove of crushed garlic; add 1 spring onion finely chopped; add finely diced cucumber; add any freshly chopped herb – chives, mint, parsley, tarragon and dill are particularly good; mix in a little Dijon or dried English mustard; subtly flavour with curry powder; spice with coriander, caraway seed or nutmeg.

Green Sauce

(for boiled meat, chicken, ham, cold cuts)
1 cup parsley without stems
3 anchovy fillets, washed free of salt and dried
1 clove garlic
30 ml (2 tablespoons) drained capers
1 small dill pickle
1 small onion
1 cup olive oil
45 ml (3 tablespoons) wine or cider vinegar
1 pinch of salt
freshly ground black pepper

If preparing by hand, first mix and chop the parsley, anchovy and garlic, add finely chopped onion and pickle, then the capers and other ingredients. Blend together thoroughly. If using a processor, use cutting blade, processing all ingredients except the capers, pickle and onion until well blended. Add remaining items and process only for a few seconds – otherwise you will end up with a purée.

Basic Mayonnaise

(for fish, cold meat dishes, salads)
1 cup olive oil
15 ml (1 tablespoon) wine vinegar
3 egg yolks
pinch of salt
a little white pepper

Beat the egg yolks well, add the seasoning and the vinegar and beat for another minute. Now slowly – literally drop by drop – add the oil, beating all the time until the sauce thickens. The trick to a successful mayonnaise lies in the slow and gradual absorption of the olive oil, otherwise the sauce can easily separate. It is often easier to do on a large plate than in a bowl. Should the sauce separate, it can be rescued by beating another egg yolk and gradually adding the sauce to it. Dieters should use this very sparingly – it's a treat for the family.

Recipes For Alkaline Days: Vegetables

Jacket Potatoes and Fillings

Just scrub the potatoes clean – the value of the jacket potatoes is in the skin. Prick the skin before putting in a pre-heated moderately hot oven (400°F, 200°C, gas 6) – this prevents skin splitting or the potato literally exploding. It usually takes about 40 to 50 minutes depending on the size and age of the potato. Ideally it should be soft on the inside and the skin crisp. Even on the diet you can serve a little butter, or try the following fillings:

* ✳ tomato and cucumber: combine diced tomato and cucumber with a little olive oil, season and add any herb
* ✳ mixed salad: any salad greens or vegetables can be finely chopped or grated to fill the potato together with a little olive oil
* ✳ green or red pepper: put a little olive oil in a pan, slice the peppers and allow to 'sweat' over a low heat for about 15 minutes
* ✳ mushrooms: bake mushrooms in the oven in their own juice, season with a little salt and freshly ground pepper. Chop together with a little diced tomato before filling the potato.

Oranged Turnips

450 g (1 lb) turnips
2 oranges
sea salt
freshly ground pepper
good handful parsley

Peel and thinly slice the turnips. Put into a pan with a little water, grate in the rind of the oranges, season with a little salt and pepper. Bring to the boil, then simmer for 10 to 15 minutes. Drain. Put the turnips into a baking dish, pour over the juice of the oranges and bake in a moderate oven (350°F, 175°C, gas 4) for about 5 minutes. Serve garnished with chopped parsley.

Swedes with Lemon

1 large swede
1 lemon
½ cup water
sea salt
freshly ground pepper
chopped parsley

Peel the swede and cut into small pieces. Grate the lemon. Put the swede and water into a pan. Add the rind of the lemon, salt and pepper. Bring to the boil, then simmer for about 10 minutes, by which time the stock should be reduced to almost nothing and the swedes tender. Pour in the juice of the lemon. Heat for a few minutes. Serve with a liberal topping of chopped parsley.

Cabbage Casserole

1 medium-sized cabbage
1 large onion
2 firm green apples
1 red pepper
½ cup water
sea salt
freshly ground pepper
cider vinegar

Cut the cabbage into substantial wedges. Peel and finely slice the onion. Peel, core and slice the apples. Mix all three together in a deep oven dish. Add about 15 ml (1 tablespoon) of cider vinegar to the water, season with salt and pepper and pour over the cabbage. Finely chop the red pepper and scatter over the top. Cover the casserole and bake in a hot oven (425°F, 220°C, gas 5) for 30 to 40 minutes, until the cabbage is tender but still has a crispness about it.

Braised Chicory with Marjoram
450 g (1 lb) chicory
25 g (1 oz) butter or margarine
2 tablespoons dried marjoram
sea salt
freshly ground pepper

Clean and trim the chicory – though even the battered-looking leaves are fine for cooking. Lightly smear the butter or margarine on the base of a baking dish, add the chicory in leafy layers, seasoning with a sprinkling of marjoram, salt and pepper. Bake in a moderate oven (350°F, 174°C, gas 4) for about 1 hour until the chicory is tender – though it shouldn't be allowed to go limp.

Spinach with Nuts and Sultanas
450 g (1 lb) spinach
½ cup sultanas
25 g (1 oz) chopped pine nuts
15 ml (1 tablespoon) olive oil
1 clove garlic
sea salt
freshly ground pepper

Soak the sultanas in a little hot water. Clean and clip the spinach, put into a heavy saucepan with just a sprinkling of salt. Cook for about 3 minutes, drain. (Don't cook the spinach in water – it contains enough of its own.) In a skillet heat the olive oil and add finely chopped garlic, then the spinach and season with pepper. Keep the spinach on the move with a wooden spoon. After a few minutes add the plumped up sultanas and the chopped nuts. Cover the pan and cook on a very low heat for about five minutes.

Lemon Cauliflower

1 medium-sized cauliflower
1 lemon
½ tablespoon crushed coriander
1 cup water
sea salt
freshly ground pepper
2 tablespoons chopped parsley

Remove the leaves from the cauliflower and chop it into small pieces. Break off the florets. Put in a pan with the water, season with a little salt and pepper. Boil until cauliflower is tender, but not soggy. Put the cauliflower in a dish, keeping the cooking liquid. To the liquid add the juice and grated rind of the lemon, stir in the crushed coriander. Boil for a few minutes, add the chopped parsley and pour over the cauliflower.

Braised Endives

8 endives
¼ cup water
50 g (2 oz) butter or margarine
sea salt
freshly ground pepper

Arrange endives in a shallow dish, if big they should be sliced vertically in half. Melt the butter or margarine, pour over the endives and season with salt and pepper. Add the water, cover. Bake in a moderate oven (350°F, 175°C, gas 4) for 30 to 40 minutes, until they are tender but still retain some crispness. For serving, they can be garnished with grated nutmeg or a little chopped parsley.

Braised Onions

8 medium-sized onions
½ cup water
3 tablespoons sultanas
2 tablespoons crushed pine nuts
1 teaspoon dried thyme or 2 fresh sprigs
a little butter or margarine
sea salt
freshly ground pepper

Peel and quarter the onions. Arrange in a casserole dish together with all the other ingredients topped with a few dabs of butter. Cover and bake in a moderate oven (350°F, 175°C, gas 4) for about an hour.

Leek and Tomato Casserole

6 leeks
6 medium-sized tomatoes
1 lemon
12g (½ oz) butter or margarine
2 garlic cloves, crushed
sea salt
freshly ground pepper

Clean and slice the leeks crosswise. Remove the skin and seeds from the tomatoes – a quick dip in boiling water makes this easier. Arrange the chunks of leeks and the tomatoes in a casserole dish, season the layers with garlic, the juice from a lemon, pepper and very little salt. Sprinkle the top with the grated rind of the lemon; add a meagre dab of butter or margarine. Bake for 30 to 40 minutes at 350°F (175°C, gas 4).

Celery Casserole
1 large head celery
4 medium-sized tomatoes (or 1 can of plum tomatoes)
8 black olives, chopped
1 garlic clove, crushed
15 ml (1 tablespoon) olive oil
1 tablespoon pine nuts
sea salt

Clean the celery, chop into chunks. If using fresh tomatoes, drop into boiling water for a minute, drain and remove skins and seeds; if using canned tomatoes check there are no seeds or bits of skin. Heat the olive oil in a heavy pan, add the garlic and cook for a minute, add the celery then the tomatoes, finally the chopped olives and the crushed pine nuts (these are optional). Season with just a little salt. Transfer to a casserole dish and bake in a moderate oven (350°F, 175°C, gas 4) for about half an hour.

Lemon Mushrooms
450 g (1 lb) cultivated mushrooms
2 lemons
1 teaspoon dried thyme or 2 fresh sprigs
sea salt
freshly ground pepper
1 tablespoon chopped parsley

Wash and trim the mushrooms, don't peel. Put in a pan together with the juice and grated rind of the lemons, the thyme and seasonings. Cook over a low heat for a couple of minutes, stir in the parsley and simmer gently for 5 minutes. Mushrooms cook very quickly and should be done just to tenderness otherwise they can become tough and not so tasty.

Runner Beans with Sage

450 (1 lb) runner beans
1 garlic clove
1 tablespoon chopped or powdered dried sage
15 ml (1 tablespoon) olive oil
sea salt
freshly ground pepper

Trim the beans and cut them into medium-sized diagonal slices. Heat the oil in a heavy pan, add the garlic clove either finely chopped or crushed. Stir in the sage and allow the herb to penetrate the oil for a couple of minutes. Stir in the beans, add enough water for simmering (about ½ cup) and season with pepper and a little salt. Bring water to the boil, then reduce heat. Cover and allow to simmer for 5 to 7 minutes. The beans must retain a certain degree of crispness.

Mediterranean Green Beans

450 g (1 lb) runner or French beans
2 medium-sized onions
1 small can plum tomatoes
1 garlic clove
30 ml (2 tablespoons) olive oil
1 teaspoon dried oregano
sea salt
freshly ground pepper

Clean, top and tail the beans, cut into medium-sized diagonal slices if too large. Peel and chop the onions. Heat the oil in a heavy pan, add the clove of garlic finely chopped, then the onions. Cook for a few minutes; add the tomatoes (check there is no skin or pips otherwise the dish becomes acid), the oregano, a little salt and a liberal amount of freshly ground pepper. Stir to break up the tomatoes thoroughly. Simmer for 3 to 5 minutes. Add the beans. Cook over a low heat for about 10 minutes – the beans should retain some crispness. They can be served with a sprinkling of parsley.

Spicey Okra

450 g (1 lb) okra
1 onion
1 small can plum tomatoes
1 garlic clove
1 lemon
15 ml (1 tablespoon) olive oil
1 teaspoon crushed coriander
sea salt
freshly ground pepper

Wash and cut off the tails of the okra. Peel and finely chop the onion. Heat the olive oil in a heavy pan, add the onion and garlic (crushed or chopped), sauté for a few minutes. Check to see there is no skin or seeds in the tomatoes, put them in the pan, stirring to break up the tomato pulp. Add the coriander and the juice of the lemon. Season with salt and pepper. Simmer for 5 to 8 minutes, until the mixture looks like a sauce. Put in the okra. Cover and simmer for 8 to 10 minutes. Serve garnished with the grated rind of the lemon.

Lemon Courgettes (Zucchini)

6 good-sized courgettes
2 lemons
1 tablespoon chopped fresh rosemary (or thyme)
handful of chopped parsley
sea salt
freshly ground pepper

Wash and slant-slice the courgettes. Mix together with all the herbs, including a little salt and pepper. Arrange the courgettes in layers in a casserole dish, covering each with a sprinkling of the herb mixture, plus a little grated lemon rind. Pour the juice o the 2 lemons over the courgettes. Bake in a moderate oven (350°F, 175gC, gas 4) for 20 to 30 minutes.

Baked Aubergine (Egg Plant) with Rosemary

2 large aubergines
2 medium-sized tomatoes
1 onion (peeled and cut into rings)
3 cloves garlic, crushed
1 tablespoon chopped fresh rosemary, or 1 teaspoon dried
1 tablespoon chopped parsley
15 ml (1 tablespoon) olive oil
sea salt
freshly ground pepper

Slant-slice the aubergines. Sprinkle with a little salt and leave for an hour, this draws out the excess water. Rinse under cold water and dry on kitchen paper. Drop the tomatoes in boiling water for a minute, then peel and seed them, cutting them into segments. In a casserole arrange the slices of aubergines, rings of onions and tomatoes, seasoning each layer with garlic, chopped rosemary, chopped parsley and a little salt and pepper. Sprinkle the olive oil over the top. Bake for about 45 minutes in a moderate oven (350°F, 175°C, gas 4).

Stuffed Aubergines (Egg Plant)

4 large aubergines
1 cup cooked brown rice
2 garlic cloves, crushed
10 black olives, chopped
a few capers
2 tablespoons chopped parsley
30 ml (2 tablespoons) olive oil
sea salt

Cut the aubergines in half, crosswise. Scoop out about half the flesh and chop into small pieces. Cook the rice and add the chopped aubergines, olives, capers and parsley. Season with a little sea salt. Fill the aubergine shells with stuffing, cover with some olive oil, and bake in a moderate oven (350°F, 175°C, gas 4) for about an hour.

Spiced Marrow Casserole

1 small marrow – about 680g (1½ lb)
4 medium-sized tomatoes (or 1 can of plum tomatoes)
1 onion
* clove garlic*
1 teaspoon crushed coriander seeds
1 tablespoon chopped fresh basil
15 ml (1 tablespoon) olive oil
sea salt
freshly ground pepper

Peel the marrow. Cut in half and take out the seeds, then cut into smallish cubes. If using fresh tomatoes, put in boiling water for a couple of minutes in order to remove the skins easily, quarter and remove seeds. Check there are no bits of skin or seeds if canned tomatoes are used. Peel and slice the onion. Heat the olive oil in a heavy pan, add the garlic – crushed or chopped – then the onion and cook until the onion is softened, but not browned. Add the tomatoes. Stir for a few minutes, then take off the heat. Stir in the diced marrow, season with a little salt and pepper. Put everything into a casserole dish, sprinkle with coriander and finely chopped basil. Cover and bake in a moderate oven (350°F, 175°C, gas 4) for 40 to 50 minutes. The marrow will produce considerable liquid, so drain before serving or reduce the liquid over a hot flame for a few minutes.

Stuffed Peppers

4 firm green peppers
150 g (6 oz) brown rice
1 cup water
2 medium-sized onions
4 medium-sized tomatoes
2 garlic cloves, crushed
8 black olives, chopped
1 tablespoon fresh rosemary or thyme (½ teaspoon dried)
1 tablespoon freshly chopped parsley
sea salt
freshly ground pepper

Bring to the boil 1 cup water, add the brown rice and simmer for about 30 minutes. Do not salt. Drop the tomatoes into boiling water, skin and seed them by cutting into quarters. Peel and dice the onion. In a bowl, mix together the rice, tomatoes, onions, garlic, olives, herbs and seasoning. If this appears very dry, add a little olive oil. Clean and cut the tops off the green peppers, also remove the pips and the pith. Stuff each pepper with the rice mixture – put a little olive oil on the top. Put in a baking dish, cover with foil and bake in a moderately hot oven (425°F, 220°C, gas 5) for about 30 to 40 minutes.

Green Pepper and Onion

3 green peppers
2 medium-sized onions
1 clove garlic, crushed
30 ml (2 tablespoons) olive oil
1 dessertspoon dried dill
sea salt
freshly ground pepper

Wash and seed the peppers, removing the pith as well. Cut into strips. Peel and slice the onions. Put the oil in a heavy pan; heat. First add the garlic for a few seconds, then the peppers and onions, mingling them well. Season with a little salt and some freshly ground pepper. Cover and steam over a low heat for 7 to 10 minutes until peppers are tender. Add the dill. Steam for another few minutes.

Ratatouille

6 courgettes (zucchini)
2 aubergines (egg plant)
4 tomatoes
1 green pepper
2 medium-sized onions
1 garlic clove
15 ml (1 tablespoon) olive oil
1 teaspoon dried oregano or marjoram
sea salt
freshly ground pepper

Peel and dice the onion. Wash and cut the courgettes into circular slices. Wash and cut the aubergines into smallish chunks. Wash and cut the pepper into slices, taking away the seeds and white pith. Drop the tomatoes into boiling water for a few minutes, peel, seed and cut into quarters. Heat the oil in a heavy pan, add the garlic – crushed or very finely chopped – stir with a wooden spoon and add the oregano or marjoram, put in the tmatoes and cook for a minute. Add the onions, green pepper, courgettes and aubergines; season with a little salt and pepper. Cover and cook over a very low heat for 20 to 30 minutes – stirring from time to time – until the vegetables are tender.

Recipes For Alkaline Days: Soups

Basic Vegetable Soup

1 cup chopped onions
3 stalks celery, chopped
2 medium-sized potatoes, chopped
4 carrots, chopped
6 cups water
1 cup of any chopped root vegetable
2 cups coarsely chopped leafy vegetable (cabbage, spinach, broccoli, etc.)
sea salt
freshly ground pepper

Put a smear of olive oil into a large pan, sauté the onions and celery just a little. Add the other vegetables, cover with water, season with a little salt and ample ground pepper (a few whole peppercorns can also be added). Bring to the boil, lower the heat and simmer for 30 minutes. Now add the leafy vegetables and cook for a further 3 to 5 minutes.

Onion and Potato Soup

2 medium-sized onions
3 medium-sized potatoe
6 cups water
grated nutmeg
sea salt
freshly ground pepper
chives or parsley for garnishing

Chop the onions, dice the potatoes, cover with the water and boil until tender (about 15 to 20 minutes). Now season with a mere flick of salt, some freshly ground pepper and a little grated nutmeg. Put through the blender and serve garnished with chives or parsley. This soup can easily be converted into a zesty curry soup by stirring in some curry powder (about two teaspoons) before liquidising.

Garlic Soup

2 heads of garlic
25g (1 oz) butter
15 ml (1 tablespoon) olive oil
6 cups vegetable stock (cooking water from any vegetable)
2 medium-sized potatoes
pinch of sage
sea salt
freshly ground pepper

Peel the garlic cloves and finely chop, then sauté in the combination of butter and oil – be careful not to burn it. Heat the vegetable stock and pour over the garlic; season with a little salt and pepper. Simmer for about 15 minutes. Peel and dice the potatoes and add to the pot, cooking for a further 15 minutes or until the potatoes are done, flavouring first with a pinch of powdered sage. Put through the blender.

Continental Green Bean Soup

1 onion
2 leeks (or another onion)
15 ml (2 tablespoons) olive oil
4 medium-sized potatoes
450 g (1 lb) green string beans
2 tomatoes
6 cups water
sea salt
freshly ground pepper

Chop the onion and leeks and sauté in the olive oil until soft. Peel and dice the potatoes, trim and slice the beans into medium-sized pieces. Skin and seed the tomatoes (first dip them in boiling water) and cut into pieces. Add everything to the onion and leeks, cover with the water. Simmer for about 30 minutes. Flavour to taste with not that much salt, but a liberal amount of pepper.

Hot Cucumber Soup
1 medium-sized cucumber
1 medium-sized potato
1 onion
3 to 4 cups of water
12 g (½ oz) butter
sea salt
freshly ground pepper

Chop the onions, peel the potatoes and cucumber, then grate both of them. Put enough butter in a heavy pan just to grease it, put in onions, cucumber and potatoes and allow them to 'sweat' together over a very low heat. This takes only about 5 minutes. Heat the water to just boiling point, pour into the pan and simmer the soup for 20 minutes. Now season with salt and pepper to taste. This soup can either be served as it is, or put through the blender. It looks and tastes particularly good if a little yoghurt is stirred in at the last minute.

Carrot Soup with Orange
900 g (2 lb) carrots
2 small onions
1 medium-sized potato
25 g (1 oz) butter
3 cups water
1 orange
sea salt
freshly ground pepper
chopped parsley

Chop the onion into small pieces and sauté over a low heat in the butter. Brush and clean the carrots, keeping on as much skin as possible; slice. Add the carrots to the onions and stir around so they are covered with the butter, and cook over a low heat for about 5 minutes. Peel and quarter the potato and add to the pot. Cover with about 3 cups of water, bring to the boil and continue at a moderate bubbling for about 20 minutes.

The potato cooks fairly quickly, but check the carrots. Season withsalt and pepper. Put through a liquidiser. This usually makes quite a thick pureé and may need a litle water to thin it down. Grate the rind from the orange, put aside. Juice the orange and add it to the soup just before serving. Sprinkle the grated peel on the top together with a little chopped parsley.

Cauliflower Soup

2 medium-sized onions
1 large cauliflower
2 green cooking apples
2 carrots
½ lemon
grated nutmeg
sea salt
freshly ground pepper
chopped parsley

Peel and slice the onions, apples and carrots. First boil the onions and carrots, but don't salt them, then for the last 5 minutes add the apples, quartered. In a separate pan, lightly cook the cauliflower, using a few of the green leaves along with the florets. Drain, retain the cooking liquids fom both pots. Liquidise all the vegetables using the liquid to regulate desired thickness. Return to one pan, add the juice of ½ lemon and a little grated nutmeg. Season with salt and pepper. Before serving, garnish with chopped parsley.

Spinach Soup

2 medium-sized onions
900g (2 lb) spinach
1 lemon
grated nutmeg
sea salt
freshly ground pepper

Peel and slice the onions, boil until tender. Cook the spinach in very little water and for only a few minutes. Liquidise the two together; return to one pan. Add water to adjust thickness, also the grated rind and juice of a lemon, a little grated nutmeg and season with salt and pepper.

Mushroom Soup

3 medium-sized onions
450 g (1 lb) mushrooms
1 carrot
sea salt
freshly ground pepper

Peel and chop the onions. Wash and stalk the mushrooms, keeping the stalks and putting them together with half the mushroom caps and the onions into a pan with very little water. Simmer until soft. Put through the blender. Meanwhile chop the remaining mushroom caps into small pieces. Put the pureé in a pan, add a little water, season with salt and pepper, then add the chopped mushrooms. Simmer just enough to soften the mushrooms.

Recipes For Alkaline Days: Sauces

Quick Tomato Sauce

(to pour over vegetable casseroles for additional liquid and taste)
30 ml (2 tablespoons) olive oil
1 clove garlic
1 medium-sized onion
15 ml (1 tablespoon) tomato pureé
1 400-g (14-oz) can Italian plum tomatoes
little salt
freshly ground pepper

Finely chop the garlic clove and sauté in heated olive oil; be careful not to burn it. Add finely chopped onions and cook until soft. Add the tomato pureé, stirring well with a wooden poon. Add the tomatoes, making sure that no skin or pips go into the sauce (otherwise it is an acid food). Simmer the sauce over a very low heat for 20 to 30 minutes, stirring from time to time; if the reduced sauce is too thick, simply add a little water.

Finally season with a little salt and freshly ground pepper.

You can alter the character of this basic sauce by adding herbs: parsley, thyme or oregano are good, so is freshly chopped basil added at the last minute; interesting too is tarragon, which can be used dry – 30 ml (2 tablespoons) should be simmered in with the sauce. A tasty hot sauce is made by sautéing a little finely chopped chilli pepper with the garlic – but go easy, it's very strong and you need only the smallest amount, and discard the pips; a final addition of coarsely chopped basil provides a cool contrast.

Raw Tomato Sauce

(As a relish for vegetable dishes)
6 medium-sized tomatoes
½ cup finely chopped shallots
1 clove garlic, finely chopped
30 ml (2 tablespoons) olive oil
good handful of freshly chopped basil
salt and freshly ground pepper

Peel the tomatoes and remove the pips, cut into small pieces. Put all the ingredients except the seasoning in a blender and process until it is almost a pureé. Finally, season to taste.

Soya Mayonnaise

(an alternative without eggs for limited salad use)
1 cup olive oil
50 g (2 oz) soya flour
90 ml (6 tablespoons) water

This is the alkaline substitute for regular mayonnaise. Mix the soya flour and water to a smooth paste, and then slowly add the oil drop by drop, beating all the time until it starts to thicken, then the oil can be added at a faster rate, though it should not be poured in. This sauce can also be used on acid days.

Recipes For Salad Mixers

Coleslaw with Fruit and Yoghurt

225 g (½ lb) cabbage
1 carrot
2 firm green apples
small bunch green grapes (optional)
½ lemon
1 small carton natural yoghurt
sea salt
freshly ground pepper

Clean and shred the cabbage. Peel and grate the carrot. Peel and finely slice the apples. If grapes are used, seed and slice them. Toss together the cabbage, carrots, apples and grapes. Mix together in a bowl the yoghurt, seasoning, juice and rind of the lemon. Pour the dressing over the cabbage, carrot, apples and grapes. A sprinkling of crushed pine nuts is a good extra garnish.

Caraway Cabbage

½ medium-sized red cabbage
½ small green cabbage
1 onion
1 garlic clove, crushed
30 ml (2 tablespoons) olive oil
15 ml (1 tablespoon) cider or wine vinegar
1 teaspoon caraway seeds
sea salt
freshly ground pepper

Shred or very finely slice the cabbages. Peel and chop the onion nto very small pieces. Combine the three. Make the dressing – crushed garlic, olive oil and vinegar, seasoned with very little salt, pepper – and finally add the caraway seeds. Pour the dressing over the cabbage salad and mix in well. Allow to marinate for at least half an hour before serving.

Spinach Salad
(if eaten on aid days, also 2 rashers of lean bacon)
450 g (1 lb) spinach
handful of button mushrooms
1 lemon
sea salt
freshly ground pepper

Wash and stalk the spinach. Wash and finely slice the mushrooms. In a small bowl, mix together the juice and rind of the lemon, a little sea salt and pepper. Toss together. On acid days, sauté the bacon in a heavy pan with no extra fat, cut into small pieces and after absorbing excess fat on kitchen paper, sprinkle over the salad.

Tomato Salad
6 ripe tomatoes
3 spring onions or 1 tablespoon chopped chives
1 tablespoon chopped parsley or fresh basil
sea salt
freshly ground pepper
a little olive oil

Clean and slice the tomatoes. Chop the onions or chives into very small pieces. Arrange on a plate, season with a minimum amount of salt, a little fresh pepper and a covering of olive oil and a garnish of parsley or basil.

Raw Onion Salad

3 or 4 medium-sized onions
2 medium-sized tomatoes
45 ml (3 tablespoons) olive oil
15 ml (1 tablespoon) cider or wine vinegar
½ teaspoon dried oregano
2 tablespoons chopped parsley
sea salt
freshly ground pepper

Peel and slice the onions into thin circles. Thinly slice the tomatoes. Arrange on a platter in alternating layers. Mix the dressing by combining the oil, vinegar and oregano, plus a little salt and pepper to taste. Finally add the parsley. Pour over the salad and allow to marinate in the refrigerator for a minimum of half an hour before serving.

Carrot and Orange Salad

4 to 5 large carrots
1 box mustard and cress
1 orange
½ lemon
30 ml (2 tablespoons) olive oil
1 tablespoon chopped parsley

Mix together the oil, juice and rind of both the orange and ½ lemon, season with very little salt. Clean and grate the carrots, snip the stems off the cress. Mix the two together, pour over the dressing and garnish with a sprinking of very finely chopped parsley.

Fennel Salad

2 medium-sized fennel bulbs
½ cucumber
1 tomato
½ lemon
½ small carton natural yoghurt
sea salt
freshly ground pepper

Clean and slice fennel into small sections. Peel and dice the cucumber and mix in with the fennel. Make the dressing by combining the yoghurt, juice and rind of the lemon, a little salt and pepper. Pour the dressing over the salad, making sure the vegetables are well covered. Chop the tomato into very small pieces and toss on top.

Chicory and Citrus Salad

1 large chicory head
1 bunch watercress
2 oranges
1 lemon
30 ml (2 tablespoons) olive oil
45 ml (3 tablespoons) cider or wine vinegar
sea salt
freshly ground pepper
a little mustard powder

Wash the chicory and break into bite-size pieces. Clean and top the watercress. Take the rind from the oranges and slice into thin rings. Grate the rind from the lemon and juice the remaining fruit. Put the chicory, watercress and orange slices in a bowl, toss well. Make a dressing from the olive oil, vinegar, juice of lemon, little salt and pepper and a touch of mustard powder. Mix very well, pour over the salad. The salad may be garnished with crushed sunflower or sesame seeds.

Radish Salad

20 radishes
1 garlic clove, crushed
1 tablespoon finely chopped parsley
1 tablespoon chopped chives or spring onions
30 ml (2 tablespoons) olive oil
15 ml (1 tablespoon) lemon juice
sea salt
freshly ground pepper

Wash, top and tail the radishes. Cut into very thin slices. For the dressing, mix together the olive oil, lemon juice, crushed garlic clove, chives or spring onions with a little salt and pepper. Add to the radishes, mix well and garnish with parsley.

Raw Beetroot Salad

3 uncooked beetroot
1 firm green apple
2 sticks celery
60 ml (4 tablespoons) natural yoghurt
½ lemon
1 tablespoon desiccated coconut
sea salt
freshly ground pepper

Peel and grate the beetroot. Peel and cut the apple into small pieces. Clean and chop the celery into small chunks. Combine all together. Combine the yoghurt with the juice and rind of lemon, season lightly. Pour over the salad and garnish with a little coconut.

Spicey Courgette (Zucchini) Salad

450 g (1 lb) small courgettes
4 tablespoons chopped spring onions
1 red pepper, chopped
2 tablespoons chopped parsley
10 black olives, chopped
½ tablespoon oregano
15 ml (1 tablespoon) olive oil
2.5 ml (½ teaspoon) cider or wine vinegar
5 ml (1 teaspoon) honey melted in a little hot water
sea salt
freshly ground pepper

Wash and slice the courgettes into rings, pop into boiling water and cook for about 5 minutes. Don't salt. Drain and cool. Mix together chopped onions, red pepper, parsley and oregano. Make the dressing from oil, vinegar, honey, a little salt and pepper. Pour over the salad and toss well. Garnish with chopped black olives.

Cucumber with Yoghurt

1 large cucumber
1 garlic clove, crushed
1 cup natural yoghurt
½ lemon
1 tablespoon chopped fresh mint
sea salt
freshly ground pepper
a few lettuce leaves

Wash and finely slice the cucumbers, don't peel. Make the dressing from the yoghurt, garlic, juice from the lemon, a little salt and pepper and blend well. Pour over the cucumbers. Place salad on a bed of lettuce leaves, garnish with chopped mint and grated lemon rind.

Mushroom Salad

225 g (½ lb) button mushrooms
½ lemon
15 ml (1 tablespoon) olive oil
sea salt
freshly ground pepper

Wash and thinly slice the mushrooms including the stems. Pour over the mixture of oil, juice of lemon, a little salt and pepper. The flavour is enhanced if left for a minimum of half an hour before serving.

Mushroom and Watercress Salad

225 g (1 lb) button mushrooms
2 bunches watercress
30 ml (2 tablespoons) olive oil
15 ml (1 tablespoon) cider vinegar or lemon juice
2 tablespoons chopped parsley
sea salt
freshly ground pepper

Wash and trim the watercress. Break up into a bowl. Wash and finely slice the mushrooms, including the stems. Toss in with the watercress. Make the dressing from the oil, vinegar or lemon juice plus seasoning. Mix in with the salad and garnish with finely chopped parsley.

Chapter 5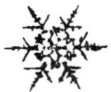

Outside Eating

A major problem with diets is how to cope with eating outside the home without the diet becoming tedious for both the dieter and other people. Of course, there are those who are so determined to stick to the prescribed nutritional path that they carry their own food with them – everywhere. Gloria Swanson was one of these; she was well known for appearing even at an official banquet with her personal meal neatly, and presumably elegantly, packaged. (Incidentally, she was a great believer in the therapeutic properties of string beans and cour gettes.) But it's the exceptional dieter who can carry off such gestures.

So how do you cope? Fortunately in the Swinging Diet there is considerable flexibility, and many of the ways of eating fall in line with the healthier attitudes towards food which are now more apparent in many eating places. The key to correct and acceptable outside eating is not only to ask for precise dishes – but to make quite sure that you get what you want. At times it is not easy, because waiters are notorious for the put-down, while assistants behind the counter at cafeterias or snack bars simply couldn't care less. So here are some guidelines on what to avoid, what to ask for and how to judge whether it is acceptable or not.

Whichever regimen you are on – acid or alkaline – the rule is to look for the simplest of dishes. This means, for a start, avoid any combination dish. The chances are that it is a mixture of acid-and-alkaline residual foods anyway, but it is also likely to be full of the worst ingredients – cheap meat or poultry with its hormone-fed hazards, hidden fat and sugar in sauces, frozen ingredients and invariably too much salt. Forget anything with a sauce – flour is out in the diet. Nothing with breadcrumbs either. And nothing fried. No soups – they

77

are nearly always made from proessed and packaged ingredients no matter how much staff swear to the contrary. Avoid chain eating places unless you can see a selection of fresh salads because practically all the main-course meals are prepared en masse, frozen then reheated in microwave ovens – all of which is bad news quite apart from the poor quality of the ingredients. And it surely goes without saying that all desserts should be avoided – and keep your hands out of the bread basket.

Salt is the real problem; in a cafeteria you can do nothing about it except avoid every single cooked dish, but in a restaurant – no matter on what level – if you are asking for a single item (such as a steak or grilled fish) it is absolutely necessary to specify *no salt* (you can always add a flicker of your own). And if it arrives obviously salted, be brave and send it back. The reaction to this is rarely good, as experience has proved, but insist; you'll be surprised what good service you can get by being difficult but knowledgeable about your request.

On Acid Days

The dieter has a slightly easier time of it during this time, because there is usually the possibility of selecting from quite a variety of dishes, but it is essential to know how to discriminate and/or give your specific requests.

At the Cafeteria or Snack Place

As mentioned before, avoid all cooked dishes. Also all cooked vegetables. For either lunch or dinner, select one of the following items and combine it with any fresh salad you can see – but a salad without any dressing on it. It is a good idea to mix up your own olive-oil-and-cider-vinegar dressing at home, put it in a small bottle that it is easy to carry and add to the naked salad. If raw vegetables are few and far between, choose instead one piece of fresh fruit from the 'mxer' list. If not available, take an apple. It is better to avoid the yoghurt in self-service places because it is rarely the natural variety.

cold cuts of beef, chicken or ham (the one time it's allowed) 2 or 3 slices

✳ 2 hard-boiled eggs – eat as little of the yolk as possible

✳ tuna fish

✳ cottage cheese (as a last resort)

✳ sardines

At the Restaurant

Here, in theory, you should be able to get exactly what you want. In practice you often have to be quite strong. Even scanning through the menu doesn't always help. It is simple to eliminate all the fancy dishes, the sauces, the obvious combinations (which cancels out almost everything) but even such straightforward items as 'poached halibut' or 'filet mignon' can present problems. It should be possible to order any simple food – though it can require some persistence. The impression is that the chef will be offended. Let him be – your body is more important than the chef's emotions.

What you need to order is a clean-cooked simple protein dish with either a salad or fresh vegetables. All this should be in every equipped kitchen. Instructions to give are: grilled, no salt and only very little butter if the food is being prepared from scratch. If it comes not as requested, complain. There is often a roast available, but look at it first. Ignore the pork, check the beef, lamb and veal. Beef should be reddish, lamb and veal, pink. Any sign of overcooking or any grey-looking meat is the clear sign not to eat it. Watch the vegetables. Ask which ones are fresh, some restaurants give honest answers, but normally the response is 'all' together with a look of offence as though frozen and canned food had still to be invented. In which case don't believe a word and settle for those on the list below. Salads can usually be relied upon, but ask to have them dressed at the table (you can hardly take your own mix) in order to control contents.

For the main dish, any of the following are good. All should be simply cooked with no salt and just a little butter or olive oil (tricky to check on this) and specify the degree of cooking. It is also necessary to specify no sauces, no embellishments, no whimseys from the kitchen.

* grilled steak of any type, cooked no further than medium/ rare
* roast beef, if rare or pink and with no fat marbling
* steak tartare without raw egg, but with tabasco sauce and capers
* roast veal if pinkish
* boiled mixed meats, but avoid sausages
* calf's liver, pinkish
* calf's kidneys
* roast chicken
* boiled chicken
* roast turkey
* grilled, baked or poached fish – any variety
* lobster, oysters and other shell fish
* fish soup
* game – land or air – rabbit, hare, venison, pheasant, grouse, pigeon etc. This is one of the best choices in many ways. It is healthy and something not likely to be indulged in at home. Take advantage
* vegetables – green leaf varieties are the most difficult to cheat on, so go for spinach – never creamed or puréed (a sign it was probably frozen), otherwise choose mushrooms, green peppers, celery
* salad – its appearance will tell you how fresh it is. The 'mixer' list covers most – just avoid any potato salad – best choice: watercress, cucumber, fennel, radishes, peppers, mushrooms, celery and tomatoes
* wine – make sure it is white and very, very dry. Wine sold

by the glass is usually not only sweet but almost always too full of sulphur as well. Stick to mineral water unless the wine is obviously a good, dry – and probably expensive – white wine

On Alkaline Days

There is not so much choice on this regimen, but then it is not so easy to be fooled. Vegetables and fruits are, after all, vegetables and fruits – both easily recognisable, though it is difficult to check on freshness. Also sugars can be sneaked into fruits – so it is best to avoid even a fruit salad and select fruit in the raw. Salt is invariably flung into the vegetables, so any precooked ones have to be avoided.

At the Cafeteria or Snack Place

Any cooked vegetable can be taken from the alkaline list, but the chances are it will have been frozen and is oversalted – but one helping a day is not going to harm. It is better to look for any raw vegetables from the alkaline and 'mixer' lists. There's also the choice of fruit – but, as mentioned above, avoid the prepared mixed fruit salad because nine times out of ten it will have been sugared. Bring your own natural yoghurt and add to freshly sliced fruit.

* any combination of salads from the alkaline or 'mixer' lists
* cooked green vegetable – one that could be fresh, such as cabbage, broccoli, spinach, carrots, courgettes, string beans
* one jacket potato with salad
* any fresh fruit

At the Restaurant

On alkaline days it is important to be selective about a restaurant. It is easier to settle for a vegetarian eating place and avoid

81

everything that has grain in it. Chinese and Eastern restaurants offer a great variety of interesting vegetable dishes, but watch out for glutinous sauces. It is usually possible to ask for a mixture of steamed vegetables if they are not on the menu. At non-Oriental restaurants, you simply have to check the vegetable list, which may mean having three starters.

* jacket potato with salad
* asparagus with lemon or butter
* artichoke vinaigrette
* avocado salad – no fish in it
* ratatouille
* any steamed, boiled or baked vegetable
* any salad
* fresh fruit

Chapter 6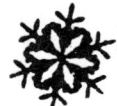

Winter Fitness: Warm Up, Slim Down

Getting into shape and keeping that way during the winter months should ideally be a three-part strategy: diet, aerobic exercise and specific body zone working. This is not so ambitious, nor so strenuous, as it might at first sound. The diet side is as outlined in detail: first the eighteen–day acid – alkaline regimen, then onto healthy intelligent eating with only a repeat of the diet after three months if necessary.

But what about exercise? It is a subject almost as controversial as diet. For every expert who makes a new claim about the benefits of a certain type of movement, there's another who says it can be bad for you. Who's got it right? The interesting thing is that when medical professionals are asked to evaluate exercise, there's a common denominator of an answer: yes to more everyday mobility, yes to certain muscle control exercises, but a big no to pushing the body too far. The current enthusiasm for running, jgging, for the exertion of rigorous aerobic work-out gets a luke-warm reception on the medical front. The respected clinics in Europe continue to take the traditional stand on exercise, using it as an integral part of any recuperation or regeneration programme, not as a health promoter in itself.

In the context of a diet, the significance of exercise lies in where the emphasis is placed; with the right programme you will help the weight move and lose inches. Too much exertion is simply not necessary – you will just be wasting your time and effort. The exercise plan orked out here should be started with the diet and then continued and ultimately made into a daily habit. It involves an awareness of how to increase mobility within the bounds of normal daily living, an effort to get outdoors for an hour a day (though 30 minutes is acceptable), and a 15-minute daily schedule to tone up the muscles of the torso.

The fundamental health benefits from exercise are that it forces more oxygen into the system and it makes the muscles work. All the other claims stem from these two basic performances. Increased oxygen turnover accelerates circulation, spurs on heart activity and boosts cellular metabolism – all of which means the efficiency of every organ is increased, whether it's the process of digestion, detoxification through the skin or the responses of the ind. Fresh air, taken calmly during a walk or even a stroll, can get the body into renewed momentum at any age. You are not losing out if you don't run, jog or take up a sport. Not all of us have athletic inclinations nor are we all capable of them. The classic cures for chronic diseases – and for just getting te body into better condition all round – still exist and still work: a gentle airing of the body in an unpolluted atmosphere, a gradual and limited exposure to the sun, a degree of rest and a graded scale of moderate exercise. You can do it all on your own without too much effort.

The first rule, then, is to get more oxygen into your body. Yogis do it simply by sitting still and breathing deeply. This has to be done outdoors – little beefit is achieved in a centrally heated dwelling. In the winter months, you need to get outside and get some fresh air into the lungs, and that means movement.

The second rule is to get the muscles going. By increasing daily activity, even to the extent of just walking more, you are going to use the long leg muscles and swing the entire body into action. The blood gets moving and is literally pumped from the feet to the heart and back again. ou are using the mass muscles of the body and burning up energy at the same time.

The third rule is to look at and assess the size of your torso. Why? Because this is where weight is most easily accumulated and most easily shifted – and that applies to both men and women. Fat is, of course, put on all over the body, but when on a diet it is the torso area which loses fat first – and without muscle toning, skin becomes slack and looks wrinkled. It is also the torso which establishes the strength, control and tone of the body. The importance of abdomen exercise has been eclipsed of late by the cult for general fitness, but it is at the very core of body culture. A most significant fact is that recent research reveals that a waist circumfrence equal to or greater than the hip measurement is a danger sign and indicates you are at higher risk for heart ailments, circulation problems and also diabetes. It is therefore important to keep trim in this area – through diet and through specific exercises. he traditional exercise-for-health regimens emphasised the importance of stomach control – through breathing, through muscles – and it is necessary once again to establish its significant place in body fitness.

Draw up a winter exercise plan that is realistic and then stick to it. It is tempting to become sluggish during the dreary weather, but once you see how the combination of the diet and the right sort of balanced exercise gives results, there's every incentive to carry on with the accommodating programme outlined here. Work on these guidelines and make a daily effort. With such a moderate – though amazingly beneficial – timetable, it is but an easy step to make it a daily habit and an obligation to keep yourself in shape. The three salient points are: move more every day, get out for an airing, learn to control your torso. Here's how . . .

Everyday Mobility

It has all been said before, but it must be repeated: whatever you can do on your own two feet, do it. Just a little more movement each day can make all the difference, whether it is walking to the shops rather than taking the car, or using the stairs rather than the lift. It seems insignificant, but it's ot. But a healthy exercise programme is not just a matter of body mobility, it is also important to gauge rest periods. Check out these points for a daily schedule:

✻ try not to sleep more than eight hours a night; many people's metabolic rate slows down considerably as though they were hibernating, so in the interests of losing weight on the eighteen-day diet or simply attaining an equilibrium afterwards, keep physically or mentally active for two-thirds of the day

✳ stay on your feet for a minimum of two hours a day, not at a stretch of course, but during everyday activities. This can be done in many ways: chores in the house or at work, shopping, walking or when on a train or bus. It is important to be vertical to aid circulation and put stress on the bones and muscles – but watch posture. Sitting down all the time is ad news for health in general, but is particularly counter-productive for the dieter

✳ think about what you could do on your own two legs without too much inconvenience. This may simply mean walking instead of taking a bus, leaving the car behind, using stairs instead of a lift, shopping at a further store. It all helps – a lot

Out in the Air

Genetically we are programmed to work on a level of oxygen established by a mobile life. This has been so for thousands of years throughout the evolution of man. Mobility outdoors was man's way of life until this century; today's life has reduced motion and contact with nature to about 10 to 15 per cent of what it was. Getting air into your lungs at a certain level of exertion is now termed 'aerobics' and many specialists have sprung up in this exercise field. Taking aerobic classes can be beneficial, but not always. Many programmes are far too ambitious, particularly for those who haven't exercised before and for those middle-aged and beyond. Less energetic – and less hazardous – regimens are perfectly rewarding, and providing you are moving out of doors for a minimum of 30 minutes a day, that is enough to keep you fit, warm you up and increase your metabolic rate. The choices within anyone's reach are:

✳ walking – the simplest way to exercise and highly recommended by all clinics. The speed at which you walk is less important than the distance. Aim for an endurance of 30 minutes of rhythmic, easy walking – you can always increase briskness as you gradually get into training. The best time is on rising and before breakfast, as your body will need to find its energy from stored fat. Do it daily. Even greater benefit comes from an additional 30 minutes later in the day – a good time is after dinner, for it not only aids digestion but can help promote a good night's sleep

* swimming – the best all-round exercise and one that is part of every clinic's regimen. It is excellent for breathing and circulation; it also builds up muscles without undue stress. Build up endurance slowly, and as with walking it is distance and time which count, not speed. Two or three weekly sessions of 30 minutes is sufficient

* cycling – this can easily become part of everyday life even during the winter months. It is great for firming the muscles of the stomach and legs. It helps heart and lungs. Speed is of no significance – aim for a methodical, continuous rhythm

* sports – skiing of course is the greatest of outdoor activities for the winter, though not all areas are blessed with the snow nor all people with the skills. Cross-country skiing, however, is for everyone and it is considered the best of all winter sports for all-round muscle use and maximum oxygen intake – and for getting a trimmer shape in record time. If there's ever the opportunity, take it

The Abdomen Shape-Up

On the eighteen-day diet you will find that abdominal fat is mobilized more easily than fat elsewhere. The purpose of these exercises is not just to help tighten the slack and provide more support for the skin, but also to help put your body at a new level of fitness. The torso muscles are the prime controllers of the body; if they are weak you don't have the sturdy framework for overall stability and undue pressure will be put on other areas of your body, in particular the back.

The area we are concerned with runs from the lower breast bone to just below the pelvis. The muscles in this area surround and protect the vital organs as well as giving support. There are three muscle groups which need to be exercised, and if you can visualise where they are, you will be more conscious of the aim of the specific movements – and more able to judge if you are doing them effectively. The main muscle group is the one that runs up the centre of the torso from the base of the pelvis to the rib cage. Called the *rectus abdominis,* it is the muscle network which tightens when the stomach is pulled up and in. Then there are the muscles high on either side of the abdomen *(transversus abdominis)* and those set at a slant at the base of the outer edges of the torso (external oblique).

Most stomach exercises usually focus on the central muscle group, but it is also important to do some twisting movements that work the two side groups and help trim that bulging area that invariably appears just below the waist, either side of the hips. The following exercises should take approximately 15 minutes; they should be performed daily and continued after the diet.

The Abdomen Effort: Women

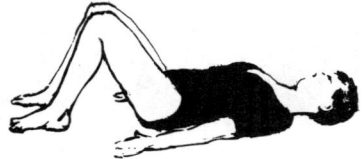 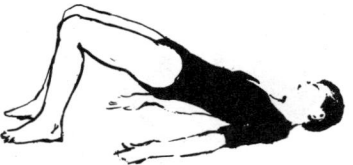

1 Lie on floor, arms at sides. Using the muscles of the stomach – no arm support – lift hips and hold to the count of five; lower slowly. Repeat 10 times

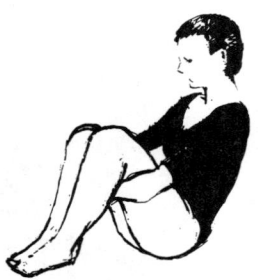 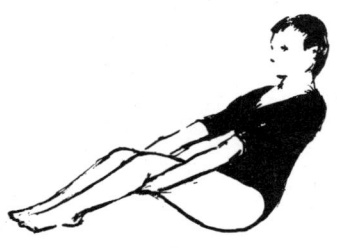

2 Sit with knees bent, arms straight in front clasping the underside of knees; roll back as far as possible and hold to the count of ten. Relax. Repeat 10 times

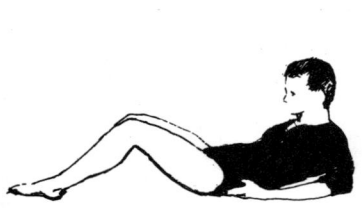 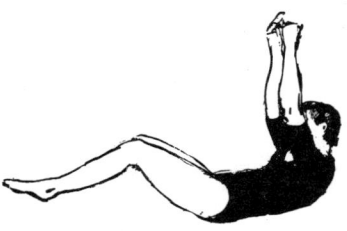

3 Lie on floor, knees bent, hands under hips with elbows supporting the torso. Raise the arms and move the pelvis upwards forcing muscles to keep it in position. Hold to the count of ten. Repeat 5 times and try to raise feet off the floor at the same time

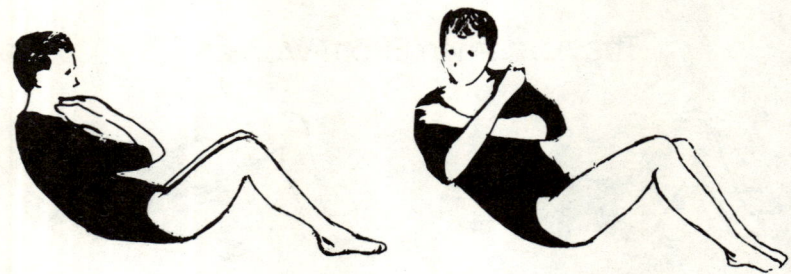

4 Sit on floor, knees bent, arms folded across chest.
Roll back, making the stomach muscles work to keep
the angle, then move the torso from side to side
holding to the count of five each side. Repeat 10 times

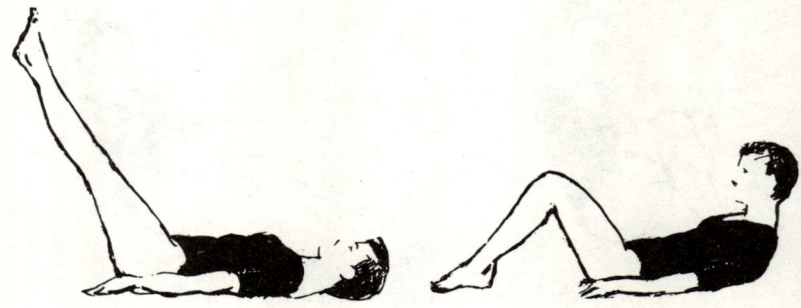

5 Lie on floor, lift both legs to an angle of 45 degrees,
arms at the sides but giving no support; raise head and
shoulders, bend knees and draw to the floor without
touching it. Hold to the count of five. Return to the
upward position. Repeat 10 times

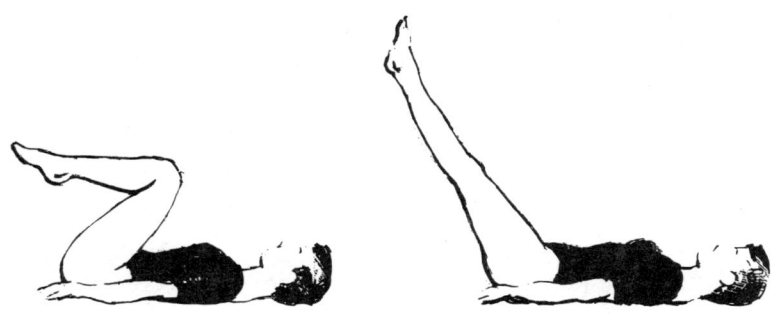

6 Lie flat on back, arms at sides but relaxed and giving
no support. Bend knees, raise to chest; slowly extend
legs and hold them straight at an angle of 45 degrees to
the count of ten. Bend legs back to chest. Repeat 10
times

The Abdomen Effort: Men

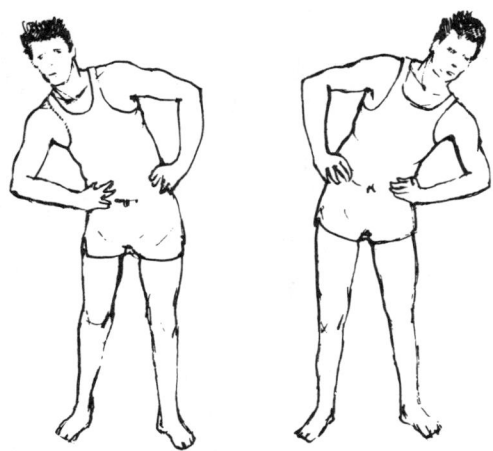

1 Stand with feet a little apart, hands on hips; move
over and bend from the seat, first to the left, then the
right, without bending over. Do 20 bends

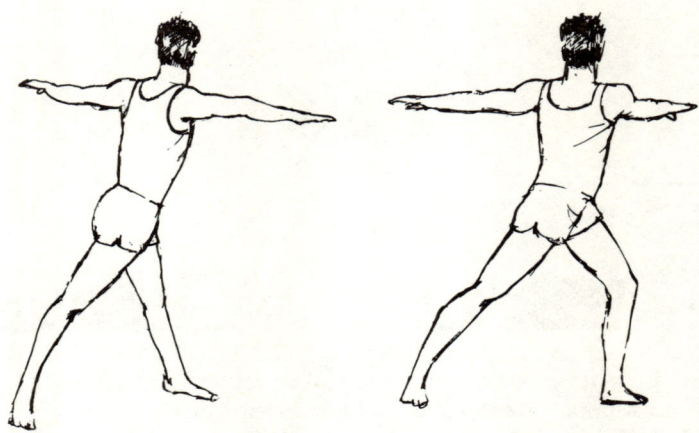

2 Stand with legs a little apart, knees relaxed, arms held in front at shoulder height. Twist the torso from the waist up only by swinging arms from one side to the other. Swing to the left and count three, to the right and count three. Repeat 20 times

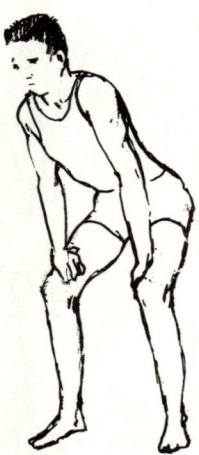

3 This is a yoga movement that does wonders for stomachs despite its simplistic approach. Stand with legs apart, knees bent. Lean over and place hands just over the knees, fingers inward. Start to breathe deeply and regularly, but independent of breathing start to contract and expand stomach muscles. In and out, in and out – you will be able to see them moving.
Continue for 2 or 3 minutes

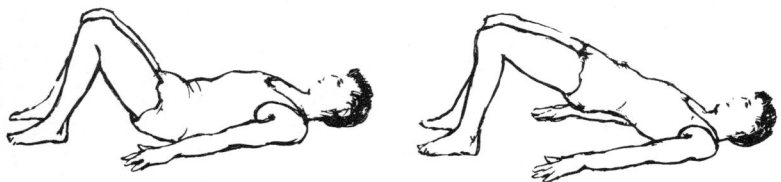

4 Lie on floor, arms at sides. Using the muscles of the
stomach – don't rely on the arms for support – lift the
hips and hold to the count of five; lower slowly.
Repeat 10 times

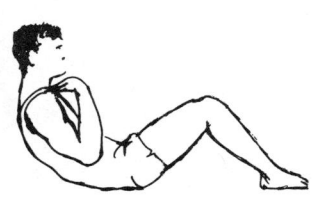 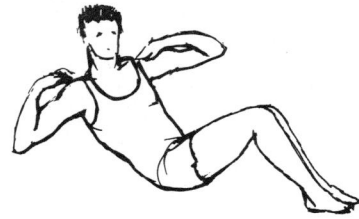

5 Lie on floor, sit up, bend legs and bring hands to
shoulders, pull and brace those muscles. Pull the body
up to a curving position, then twist from side to side,
10 times each side

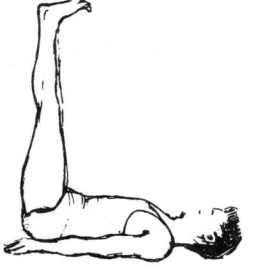 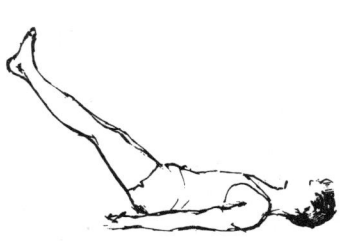

6 Lie on floor, arms relaxed at sides giving no
support. Raise legs as high as possible; hold to the
count of five, lower very slowly and don't allow to
touch the floor. Raise again and repeat 10 times

Index

96